Teen Guide to

BECOMING A MEDICAL DOCTOR

Sara Rowe Moun

ReferencePoint Press

San Diego, CA

ReferencePoint Press®

Printed in the United States

For more information, contact:
ReferencePoint Press, Inc.
PO Box 27779
San Diego, CA 92198
www.ReferencePointPress.com

LIBRARY OF CONGRESS CATALOGING-IN-PUBLICATION DATA

Names: Mount, Sara Rowe, author.
Title: Teen guide to becoming a medical doctor / by Sara Rowe Mount.
Description: San Diego, CA : ReferencePoint Press, Inc., 2025. | Includes bibliographical references and index.
Identifiers: LCCN 2024035117 (print) | LCCN 2024035118 (ebook) | ISBN 9781678210120 (library binding) | ISBN 9781678210137 (ebook)
Subjects: LCSH: Medicine--Vocational guidance--Juvenile literature. | Physicians--Juvenile literature.
Classification: LCC R690 .M684 2025 (print) | LCC R690 (ebook) | DDC 610.69/5023--dc23/eng/20240802
LC record available at https://lccn.loc.gov/2024035117
LC ebook record available at https://lccn.loc.gov/2024035118

CONTENTS

Medical Doctor at a Glance 4

Introduction 5
A Demanding Career That Is in Demand

Chapter One 9
Different Kinds of Doctors

Chapter Two 17
Becoming a Doctor: Medical School

Chapter Three 24
Becoming a Doctor: Residency

Chapter Four 32
The Day-to-Day Work of a Doctor

Chapter Five 41
What Skills and Personal Qualities Are Needed?

Chapter Six 46
Looking to the Future

Source Notes 53
Interview with a Medical Resident 55
Find Out More 58
Index 60
Picture Credits 64
About the Author 64

MEDICAL DOCTOR AT A GLANCE

Number of Jobs
As of 2022: 816,900 to 989,320, depending on the source

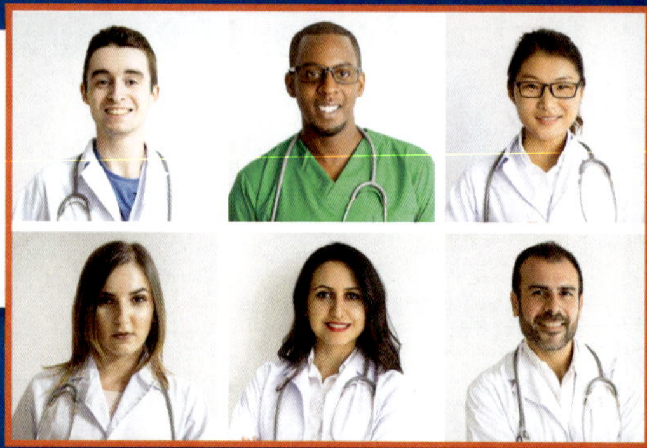

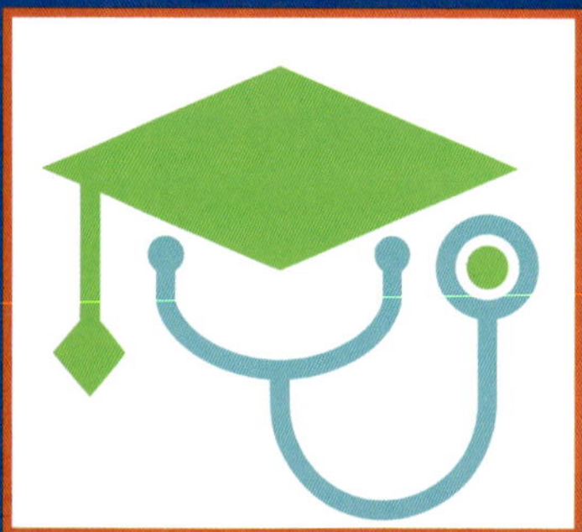

Educational Requirements
Bachelor's degree, medical school, medical residency

Certification and Licensing
State medical license required

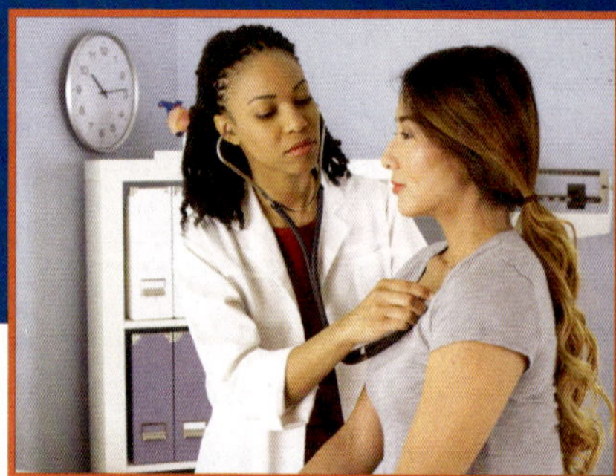

Work Settings
Hospitals, medical clinics, government agencies, nonprofit organizations, insurance companies, pharmaceutical companies

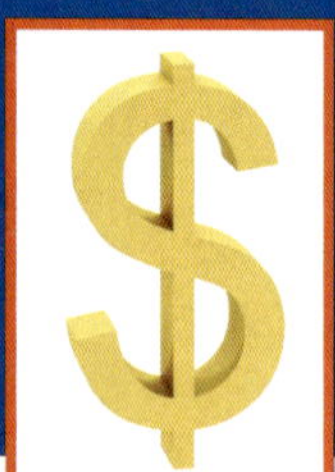

Pay
2023 median pay $239,200

Personal Qualities
Persistence, intelligence, confidence, humility, empathy

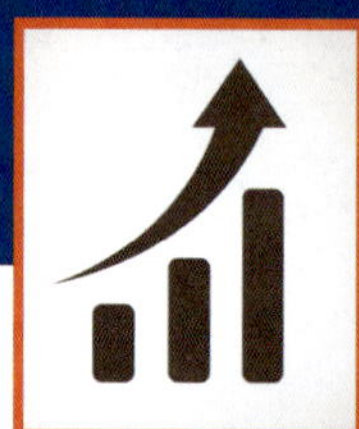

Future Job Outlook
Projected growth of 3 percent through 2032

A Demanding Career That Is in Demand

As Dr. Kevin Jubbal navigated the many years involved in medical school and then supervised hands-on experience treating patients in residency, he recognized the numerous challenges throughout the process for both him and his peers. They included long hours studying and seeing patients, low pay while in residency, and high student loans for medical school. Difficulties with life-work balance also make it a struggle to reduce stress and maintain relationships. Every day doctors also encounter patients who are sick, hurting, and sometimes difficult. Doctors might have to pass on devastating diagnoses and may not be able to find a cause for every patient's symptoms, which is frustrating both for patients and for doctors.

Jubbal founded Med School Insiders to prepare medical students for these realities so they would be better equipped to manage stress and other obstacles throughout their education and career. He is passionate about preparing future doctors to be successful in their careers because he believes that "while being a doctor is one of the most challenging and arduous careers to enter, it's truly a privilege and a tremendously rewarding profession." The personal connections made with patients is one of the most rewarding parts of the job for Jubbal. He says, "It's truly an honor to be trusted with another human being's health and wellbeing, which requires a deep level of trust. . . . As a physician, you are there for patients in their most trying times."[1]

> "While being a doctor is one of the most challenging and arduous careers to enter, it's truly a privilege and a tremendously rewarding profession."[1]
>
> —Dr. Kevin Jubbal, Med School Insiders

There is much that is appealing about the medical field. It offers the opportunity to save lives, prolong life, and improve the quality of life for patients. It also involves the use of science to develop new techniques, discover better treatment plans, and cure diseases. It is a high-paid career path that is both stimulating and challenging. Jubbal reflects, "Medicine is just a straight awesomely fascinating profession. The way the human body works, the complexities and nuances—there's just so much interesting science to uncover."[2] It also is a field in which there continues to be a high demand for new doctors.

Demand for New Doctors

Most of the demand for new doctors is created by doctors leaving the medical field. While some of these doctors are no longer practicing medicine due to pursuing other jobs, many are simply retiring due to being at or past retirement age or retiring early due to burnout. When the Physicians Foundation surveyed doctors in March 2021, a year after the onset of the COVID-19 pandemic, it found that 38 percent were considering retirement in the next year. While many doctors are getting closer to retirement, so is the general population, which also fuels the need for more doctors to treat them. "By 2035, there will be more seniors aged 65 or older than children aged 17 or younger—the first time this demographic imbalance has occurred in the nation's history," says James Taylor, president of the leadership solutions division at AMN Healthcare. "Older people see a physician at three or four times the rate of younger people and account for a highly disproportionate number of surgeries, diagnostic tests, and other medical procedures."[3]

Overall health in the United States is also impacting the need for more doctors. The Centers for Disease Control and Prevention reported in 2024 that approximately 129 million Americans suffer from chronic health conditions, including diabetes, depression, asthma, cancer, and coronary heart disease. Much of the population suffering from chronic conditions is clustered in more rural areas such as the Southeast, Maine, and the Pacific Northwest, where there is less access to medical care than in other areas of the country. Taylor says that in these areas of the country, "many patients simply don't see a physician until their problem becomes critical and they go to the emergency room. This is the least optimal method of providing care."[4]

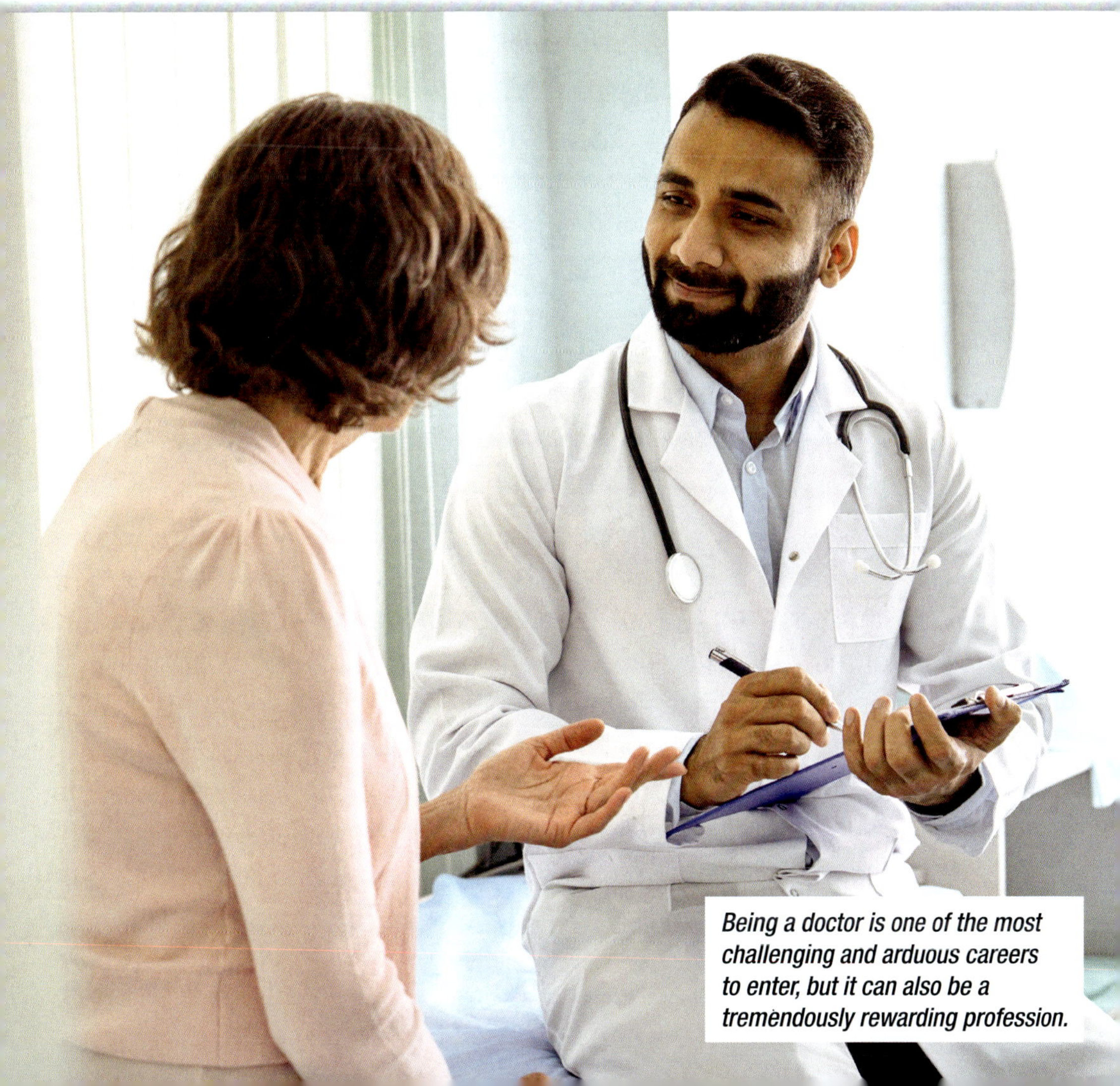

Being a doctor is one of the most challenging and arduous careers to enter, but it can also be a tremendously rewarding profession.

Where Doctors Are Needed

There are dozens of medical specialties, but the ones most in demand, according to the Doximity *2023 Physician Compensation Report*, are family medicine, psychiatry, internal medicine, emergency medicine, and obstetrics and gynecology (more commonly known as OB-GYN). The need for primary care physicians who can monitor the health of patients and diagnose conditions before they become critical or chronic is especially great. Worsening mental health, reduced stigma surrounding seeking treatment, and better diagnostic criteria have also increased the need for psychiatrists to diagnose and treat patients struggling with mental illnesses and disorders.

The areas of the country most in need of primary care or family medicine doctors are rural areas and densely populated urban areas found in many states, including Texas and California. The southeastern area of the country has the most need, especially Louisiana, Mississippi, and Virginia. The Health Resources and Services Administration (HRSA) estimates that there are currently approximately 30.5 million Americans living in medically underserved communities across the United States. To encourage students to move to these underserved communities and practice medicine, the HRSA offers scholarship and student loan repayment programs for certain specialties, including family medicine, pediatrics, OB-GYN, and psychiatry.

The Sacrifices Are Worth It

While the education process involves the commitment of four years of medical school and three to seven years of residency—and many, many stressful hours in between—it is a sacrifice that thousands of individuals make every year to become medical doctors. "It's fulfilling. It's more than any salary can pay you," says Dr. Paola Portela, who works as a pediatrician in the underserved area of Chicago where she grew up, "When I'm 80 years old and in a nursing home, what's going to matter is how I changed people."[5]

CHAPTER ONE

Different Kinds of Doctors

Prior to entering medical school, Dr. Ahmad Shatil Amin believed that the most important aspect of practicing medicine was saving and prolonging lives. However, after beginning his studies, he began to see the impact that treatments could have on the daily lives of patients as well. Now as a dermatologist, he believes he is improving the quality of life of each of the patients he treats. "The conditions that we treat . . . such as severe acne, eczema and psoriasis can often cause significant daily physical and emotional discomfort and even sometimes lead to social isolation," he says. "Everyday, we experience the satisfaction of our patients expressing their gratitude when we have been able to provide relief from the discomfort caused by their skin conditions."[6]

> "The conditions that we treat . . . can often cause significant daily physical and emotional discomfort and even sometimes lead to social isolation. Everyday, we experience the satisfaction of our patients expressing their gratitude when we have been able to provide relief from the discomfort caused by their . . . conditions."[6]
>
> —Dr. Ahmad Shatil Amin, dermatologist

The decision of which specialty to choose can be a challenging one, because every type of doctor's job is a little different. A surgeon, for example, has a very different job from a family medicine doctor. Beyond the fact that family medicine doctors will likely never set foot in an operating room (OR), their job requires much more interaction with patients, and they encounter a wide range of conditions and illnesses. Family medicine doctors and pediatricians are often people who are interested in connecting with and building trusted relationships with their patients. Surgeons are mostly interacting with the fascinating inner workings of the human body. Surgeons in various specialties can repair heart valves, remove a brain tumor, or replace a knee joint, both to save lives and to improve the quality of life for patients they operate on.

Pay and job conditions also vary widely. An emergency room (ER) doctor may work long shifts and be on call, while a dermatologist or allergist will usually have regular hours. Pay range can also vary widely based on the specialty. While family medicine doctors are often the most in demand, they are typically the lowest-paid doctors in the medical field. On the other hand, plastic surgeons and neurosurgeons typically capture the top salaries.

The following are some of the medical specialties that diagnose and treat patients currently in the United States.

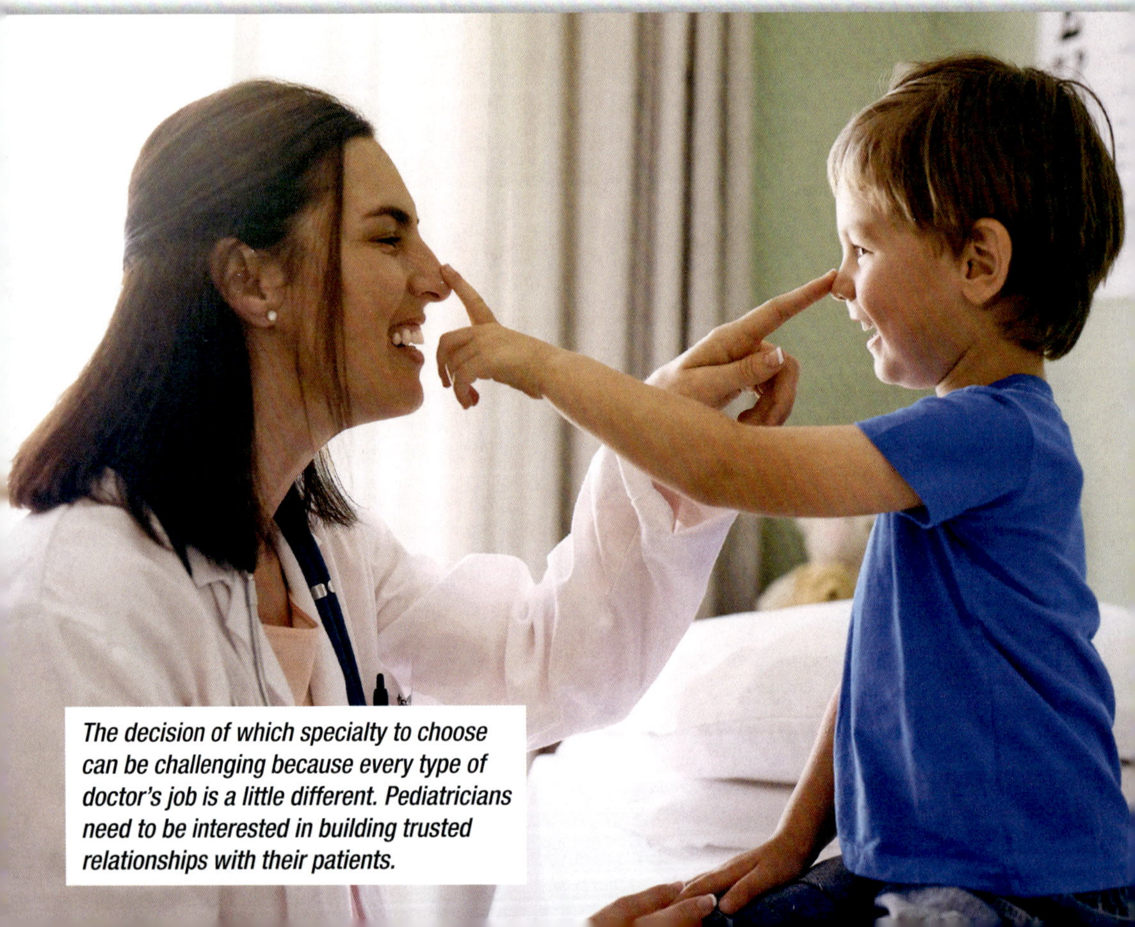

The decision of which specialty to choose can be challenging because every type of doctor's job is a little different. Pediatricians need to be interested in building trusted relationships with their patients.

Allergists

Allergists treat allergies and related immune disorders. They provide treatments for everything from seasonal allergies to asthma, chronic sinus or ear infections, and food allergies and intolerances. First an allergist will determine the source of the allergies, which may include administering skin tests, blood tests, and pulmonary function tests. Once the source of the allergic reaction is determined, an allergist will prescribe treatment. Depending on the type and severity, this may include prescribing an EpiPen, providing immunotherapy such as allergy shots, and administering intravenous immunoglobulin for immune disorders. For those with food allergies, an allergist may administer oral food tests, overseeing the gradual introduction of a small amount of the allergen with the goal of desensitizing the body until there is no immune reaction.

Anesthesiologists

Anesthesiologists specialize in providing patients with anesthesia, which will put them to sleep during surgery. Prior to surgery, they determine each patient's fitness for surgery by studying their health and test results. Their plan for anesthesia is developed with this information, since administering the correct amount of medication is dependent on factors such as the type and length of surgery, the patient's weight and health, and how they have reacted to an esthesia in the past. Prior to surgery beginning, the anesthesiologist administers anesthesia and then will monitor the patient for the entirety of the surgery. This includes monitoring vital signs and administering any blood, medications, or fluids that the patient needs. After surgery is concluded, the anesthesiologist monitors patients until they come out of sedation and determines when they can be either sent home or moved into a recovery room in the hospital.

Plastic Surgeons

Plastic surgeons have the reputation of being vanity doctors, reversing the aging process and giving people the faces and bodies

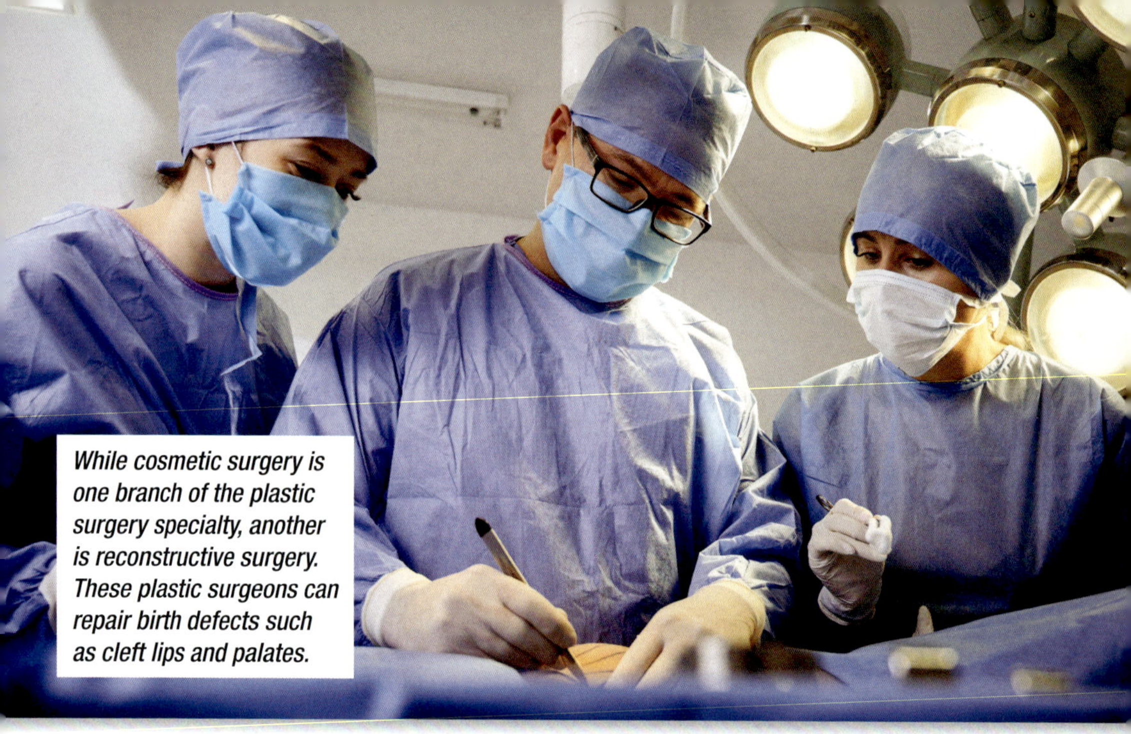

While cosmetic surgery is one branch of the plastic surgery specialty, another is reconstructive surgery. These plastic surgeons can repair birth defects such as cleft lips and palates.

they wish they had. While cosmetic surgery is one branch of the plastic surgery specialty, another is reconstructive surgery. These plastic surgeons repair birth defects such as cleft lips and palates. Plastic surgeons can also perform reconstructive surgery for damage sustained from burns, wounds, and cancer treatment. Other plastic surgeons may specialize in gender affirmation surgery for transgender individuals. Plastic surgeon Dr. Chris Homsy says, "I'm . . . most passionate about . . . providing care for transgender patients. This is something that is really necessary for patients to feel comfortable in their own skin."[7] Another appeal of this specialty is that it is one of the highest paid in the medical field, with an annual income averaging $619,000.

Cardiologists

Cardiologists are doctors that specialize in the treatment of the heart and blood vessels. They can treat preexisting cardiac problems, such as congenital heart defects, as well as conditions like high cholesterol and blood pressure, endocarditis, and coronary artery disease. When patients visit their primary care physician or the ER with symptoms of heart disease or when experiencing a heart attack, a cardiologist is the specialist who will oversee their care. Unlike cardiac surgeons, they do not perform surgeries. They do perform procedures such as cardiac catheterizations, electrocardiograms, and stress tests to diagnose and monitor heart conditions and determine treatment, which could include referral to a cardiac surgeon. The cardiology specialty is considered appealing because it offers a lower-stress work environment and an average income of $507,000.

Dermatologists

Dermatologists treat conditions that affect patients' skin, as well as the hair and nails. Common conditions they encounter include acne, warts, psoriasis, eczema, skin infections, and hair loss. They also perform biopsies to test for skin cancer, remove areas of skin cancer (unless identified as being better addressed by a plastic surgeon), and monitor for any return. Dermatologists can also perform a number of procedures in their offices to treat skin conditions, as well as for purely cosmetic reasons. These include laser therapy, which can be used for removal of everything from warts to tattoos and scars, sclerotherapy for varicose veins, and Botox injections to reduce the appearance of wrinkles. Due to the combination of flexible working hours and a high income, this is a highly desired and competitive specialty.

Family Medicine Doctors

On the lower end of the salary scale is family medicine, with an average annual salary of $249,000. Family medicine doctors are primary care physicians. They see patients for annual visits to monitor ongoing health, performing a physical examination and ordering blood work to identify any potential problems. They also treat patients experiencing everything from the flu to eczema or an infected wound. They are often the doctors who are first visited when a patient exhibits a concerning health issue. They will refer patients with more serious conditions to specialists such as a dermatologist or a cardiologist for further treatment.

OB-GYNs

An OB-GYN, or obstetrician-gynecologist, specializes in the care of the female reproductive system. These doctors provide annual exams to monitor the health of girls and women's vaginas, uteruses, and breasts. Annual exams include a physical exam and screenings for sexually transmitted infections, cancers, or other disorders. They also diagnose and treat various conditions that specifically affect female health. "On a daily basis I have the honor of helping women through things that are often unmentionable in their day-to-day lives," says Dr. Vivienne Meljen. "We break down barriers to these conversations, normalize their situation, and help them feel comfortable so that we can help them get through it and get better."[8] This specialty also cares for the health of women and their babies over the course of pregnancy

What Makes Family Medicine Special

"I love what I do, and that makes all the difference in the world. Patients can see it, and many have become dear friends. This week, in addition to receiving a couple of thank you notes, I was hugged by two patients. One was an elderly man I consoled after he lost his son in an accident, the other was a patient I helped counsel through a complex medical decision. . . . Like most weeks practicing in rural southwest Missouri, I performed a small lesion removal, managed multiple diabetics, optimized asthma . . . therapies for a number of patients, treated many cases of hypertension, . . . treated a few individuals with behavioral and mood disorders, managed complex pain. . . . I believe family medicine is the heart and soul of the medical field. It encompasses pieces of all the specialties and is the doorway by which many patients get more specialized care. . . . It's about relationships and caring for entire families across multiple generations. . . . There is an art to good bedside manner, to instilling hope, to building confidence, to providing comfort, to educating, to giving counsel and to inspiring change while tailoring treatment plans that are best suited to the patient."

—Kurt Bravata, family medicine physician

Kurt Bravata, "My Message to Students: Why Family Medicine Matters," AAFP, June 19, 2019. www.aafp.org.

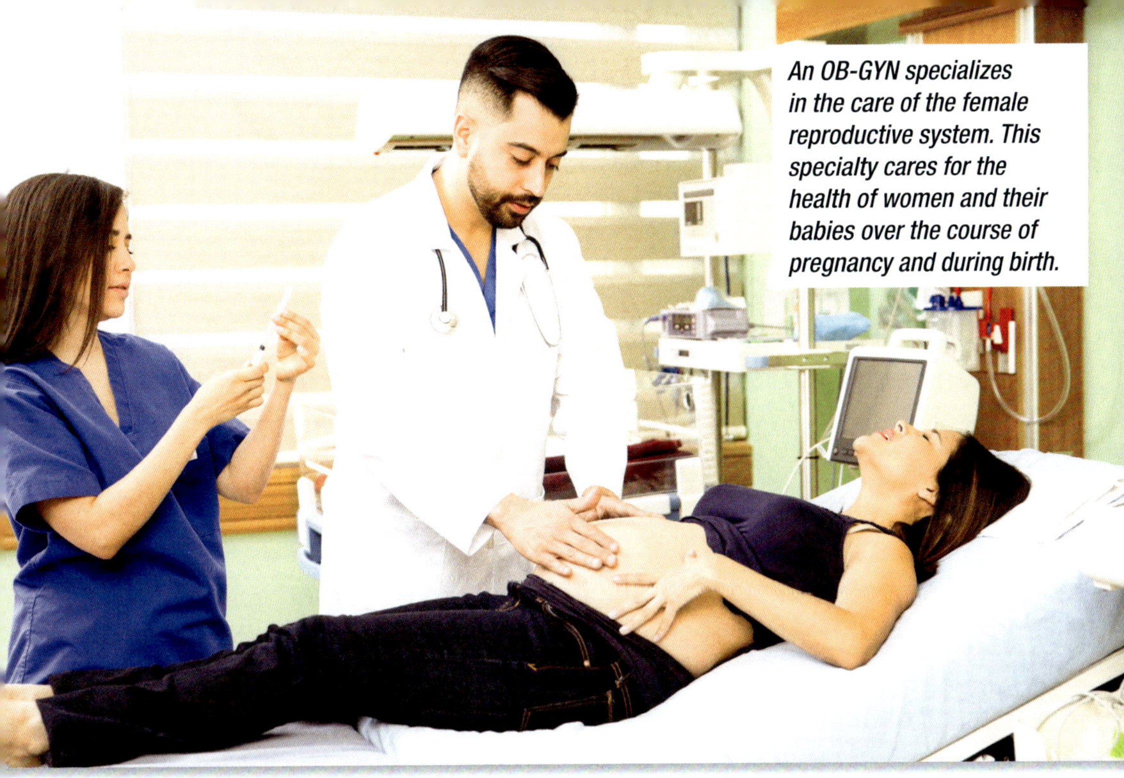

An OB-GYN specializes in the care of the female reproductive system. This specialty cares for the health of women and their babies over the course of pregnancy and during birth.

and during birth. Specialists within the field may treat infertility, women with high-risk pregnancies, and those in need of reproductive surgery.

> "On a daily basis I have the honor of helping women through things that are often unmentionable in their day-to-day lives. We break down barriers to these conversations, normalize their situation, and help them feel comfortable so that we can help them get through it and get better."[8]
>
> —Dr. Vivienne Meljen, OB-GYN

Pathologists

Pathology is one of the few medical specialties that involves little or no interaction with patients, depending on the subspeciality. Pathologists are tasked with diagnosing diseases by testing human tissue, blood, and other bodily fluids. They also spend time studying disease progression and performing research that helps the medical community better understand and diagnose diseases and conditions. Subspecialists study specific conditions, like those of the skin, blood cells, and genes or those found in children or in cases of violent or suspicious death. Blood bank/transfusion pathologists oversee the testing of blood and plasma in blood banks. While they are often the doctors who determine a diagnosis, however, the diagnoses are relayed to patients by the doctors who ordered the tests.

Rheumatologists

Rheumatologists specialize in the treatment of connective tissue, and autoimmune and inflammatory conditions, some of which can be very difficult to diagnose and treat. These conditions include arthritis, osteoporosis, lupus, tendonitis, and scleroderma. Many of these conditions cause inflammation, joint problems, fatigue, and other symptoms that affect patients' daily lives. The conditions that rheumatologists encounter are treatable but not curable and require long-term or even lifelong treatment management. They will see patients regularly to address symptoms, adjust treatment plans, and monitor progression through imaging and tests. Treatments administered include joint injections and prescribing immunosuppressants, as well as referring patients to orthopedic surgeons, physical therapists, and occupational therapists for repairs and rehab.

A Doctor for Everyone

These are only a few of the dozens of medical specialties and subspecialties currently represented in the medical field. So whether you love children or prefer interaction with test tubes instead of humans, are interested in tracking down an elusive diagnosis for struggling patients or helping teens treat their acne and feel comfortable in their skin again, with such a range of specialties that cater to different interests (and personality traits), there's likely a specialty that's the right fit for you.

CHAPTER TWO

Becoming a Doctor: Medical School

An aspiring doctor's education has only begun once his or her undergraduate studies are completed. Medical school is another four years of intensive study. But before that comes the challenging process of applying to medical school. The Association of American Medical Colleges reports that 52,577 individuals applied to medical school for the 2023–2024 school year, and 22,981 were enrolled, which is a 43.7 percent acceptance rate. Accepted students had an average 3.64 grade point average (GPA) and an average score of 506.3 on the Medical College Admission Test (MCAT). Getting into one of the top medical schools in the United States can be an even more competitive process. Harvard Medical School reports that its graduating class of 2027 has 164 students out of an applicant pool of 6,986 and an average MCAT score of 520.59 and GPA of 3.9.

Applying to Medical School

An undergraduate degree is the first requirement for application to medical school. The vast majority of students applying to medical school—30,054 of the applicants in the 2023–2024 school year—are those majoring in biological sciences. However, students majoring in the humanities, social sciences, math, and other areas also successfully apply to medical school. More important than major are the courses taken during the undergraduate years. All medical schools require applicants to have taken the following courses: chemistry (both organic and inorganic), biology, physics, and mathematics (calculus or statistics). Many schools also require an English course, biochemistry, and social science courses like sociology and psychology.

A high GPA and good grades in the required science courses are an important part of the application package. Scores on the MCAT are also key to admissions decisions. The MCAT is a computerized, standardized multiple-choice exam that tests students' knowledge in chemistry, biology, and social sciences, as well as their critical thinking skills. Total final scores range from 472 to 528.

Other parts of the application can be key to standing out among thousands of applicants with high GPAs and MCAT scores. Letters of recommendation, extracurricular activities, personal statements/essays, and at a later stage of the process, interviews are all ways to introduce admissions committees to who you are as an individual and what makes you unique among many other candidates with good test scores and grades. Dr. Kevin Jubbal of Med School

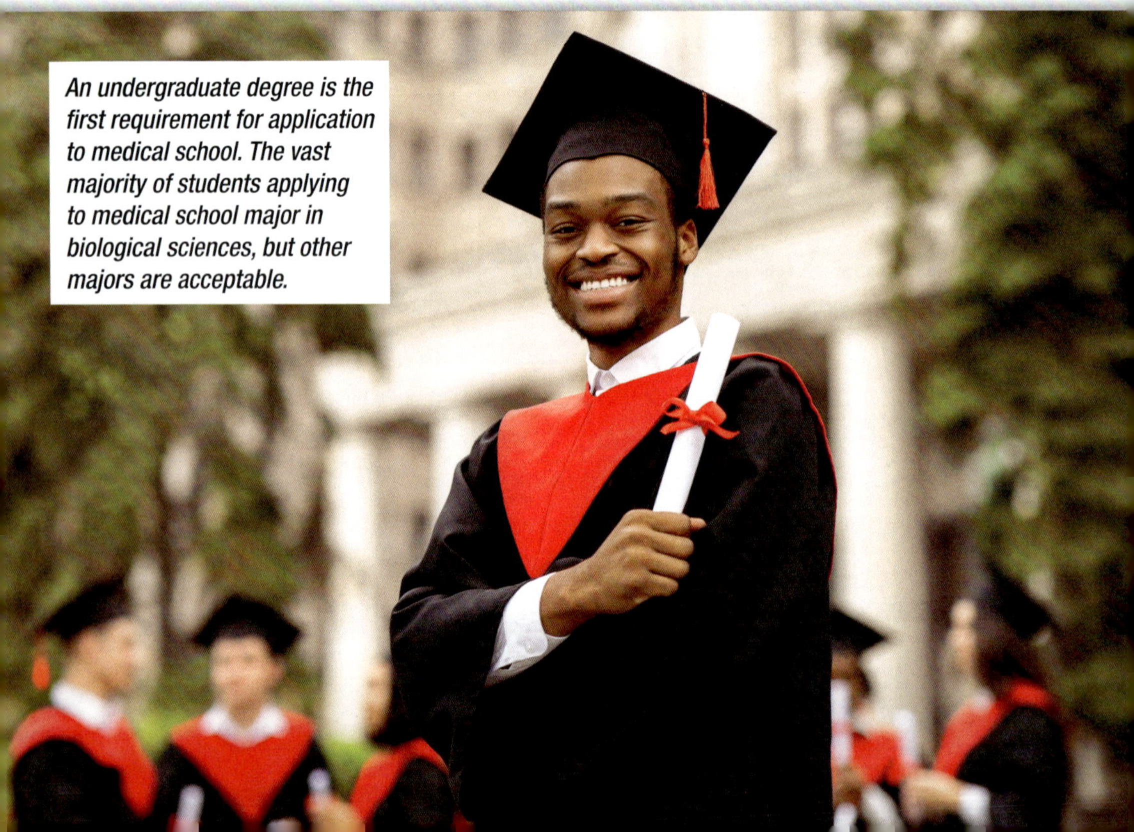

An undergraduate degree is the first requirement for application to medical school. The vast majority of students applying to medical school major in biological sciences, but other majors are acceptable.

Insiders feels that presenting themselves as well-rounded candidates is something applicants often forget: "Instead of checking boxes, you need to craft a compelling narrative. You do this by pursuing opportunities you are passionate about, which can sometimes mean diving deep into your interests outside of medicine."[9]

Just like during the undergraduate application process, it is important for students to research schools to determine safety, target, and fit. During the application process is also when students need to decide whether they would like to pursue an MD or DO degree. Medical doctors, or MDs, base their patient care on diagnosing diseases and then treating them, known as an allopathic approach. Doctors of osteopathic medicine, or DOs, focus on a model of holistic medicine, treating the body as a whole, instead of simply treating conditions. While there has been an increase in students pursuing DO degrees, in 2024 there were only 41 medical schools for DOs in the United States, compared to 159 medical schools for MDs.

Medical School Years One and Two

The transition from undergraduate school to medical school can be challenging. While there are still classes and exams, the amount of material covered and time spent studying increases, often leaving time for little else. The first two years of medical school focus on building foundational medical knowledge. Some medical schools teach from a physiological approach, in which students are first taught all the bodily systems; then pathology, or what can go wrong with these systems; and then pharmacology, or treatments. Others teach with a systems approach, which means that the physiology, pathology, and pharmacology of each system, such as the cardiovascular system, are taught individually. Learning takes place through lectures; histology labs, which involve the examination of tissues and organs; and anatomy labs, which involve cadaver dissection. First-year University of Michigan medical school student Noah Yonas says, "A lot of our time is spent in lectures. There are certain electives that we do get

"A lot of our time is spent in lectures. There are certain electives that we do get an opportunity to go to the hospital, but I think the first-year emphasis is more so just for building that foundation. And I mean, like it or not, that really does come through the classwork."[10]

—Noah Yonas, first-year University of Michigan medical school student

an opportunity to go to the hospital, but I think the first-year emphasis is more . . . for building that foundation. And I mean, like it or not, that really does come through the classwork."[10]

Lectures and labs are not the only way that students obtain that foundational knowledge, however. Another staple of the first two years of medical school is the process of patient interviews and physical exam assessments. Sometimes this involves hypothetical cases being discussed, and at other times, actors, known as standardized patients, are hired to portray patients with a certain condition or set of symptoms. Medical student Kevin Yang experienced two days a week of cases involving problem-based learning. "This consists of attempting to diagnose a hypothetical patient based on provided signs, symptoms, and labs, and concludes with the assignment of look-ups [research] based on the case," Yang says. "Every other week, we meet for Practice of Medicine sessions. . . . In these groups, led by a dynamic psychologist and physician duo, we learn patient interviewing techniques and practice our physical exam skills."[11]

While most medical schools have lectures only for the first two years, some start clinical rotations in year two. Clinical rotations take place in hospitals and clinics and allow medical students to observe and take part in the medical care of real patients while under the supervision of medical residents and attending doctors. Maggie, a University of Colorado medical student, started clinical rotations in year two of medical school, but even with parts of her day spent getting hands-on experience with patients, she still had a lot of learning (and studying) to do. Maggie says:

> After a day of attending lectures, labs, and clinical rotations, the learning doesn't stop. Although there is no traditional homework, my studying is more about reinforcing the

knowledge I gained in lectures and understanding complex medical concepts. . . . I spend every morning studying for exams. Apart from that, I sometimes have readings to complete, research to conduct, and assignments to submit.[12]

Students in both MD and DO programs also take three-part standardized exams. The first part is taken at the end of the second year of medical school as a pass/fail exam and consists of multiple-choice questions. The second part is usually taken in the fourth year of medical school, and the third is taken during residency and contains a section requiring students to examine and diagnose actors posing as patients, as well as multiple-choice questions. MD students take the United States Medical Licensing Examination, while DO students take this or the Comprehensive Osteopathic Medical Licensing Examination. These are the exams students need to take in order to become licensed doctors.

The Cost of Medical School

Medical school can require a lot of sacrifice and a lot of money. The Education Data Initiative reported in 2024 that the average yearly tuition for medical school was $58,968. This does not include books, supplies, and living expenses such as rent, transportation to school and rotations, and food. Most medical students are unable to work while attending medical school due to the heavy workload and hours spent in lectures and rotations, so most obtain large student loans. The American Association of Medical Colleges, which oversees applications to medical school and residencies, surveyed 2023 MD graduates and found they had a median $200,000 of medical school debt. Dr. Andrea Stolar, senior associate dean of student affairs at Baylor College of Medicine says, "Many people have loans. . . . Then they are going to have multi-years of residency where they are paid a salary, but not sufficiently to really start making any headway on their loans. It's a long stretch to be willing to put off the things that a lot of your friends might be doing as they start jobs and start (to) experience life."

Quoted in Sarah Wood, "How Long Is Medical School and What Is It Like?," *U.S. News & World Report*, January 12, 2024. www.usnews.com.

Medical School Years Three and Four

The majority of a medical student's time in the third and fourth year of medical school is spent rotating through different specialties. While some students may know their area of interest prior to rotations, experiencing these specialties firsthand can be key, because different types of doctors encounter different types of patients and perform different tasks in their jobs. Each clinical rotation usually lasts a month, and they sometimes require students to travel to different parts of the country for rotations in different hospitals and clinics. University of Michigan medical student Cara Ferguson found that clinical rotations resulted in her deciding to focus on pediatrics rather than her initial choice of surgery. She says, "I noticed that my head was always on a swivel when there was a pediatric patient around. I had the most fun on the pediatric rotation. My friends told me I seem[ed] the most joyful on that rotation."[13]

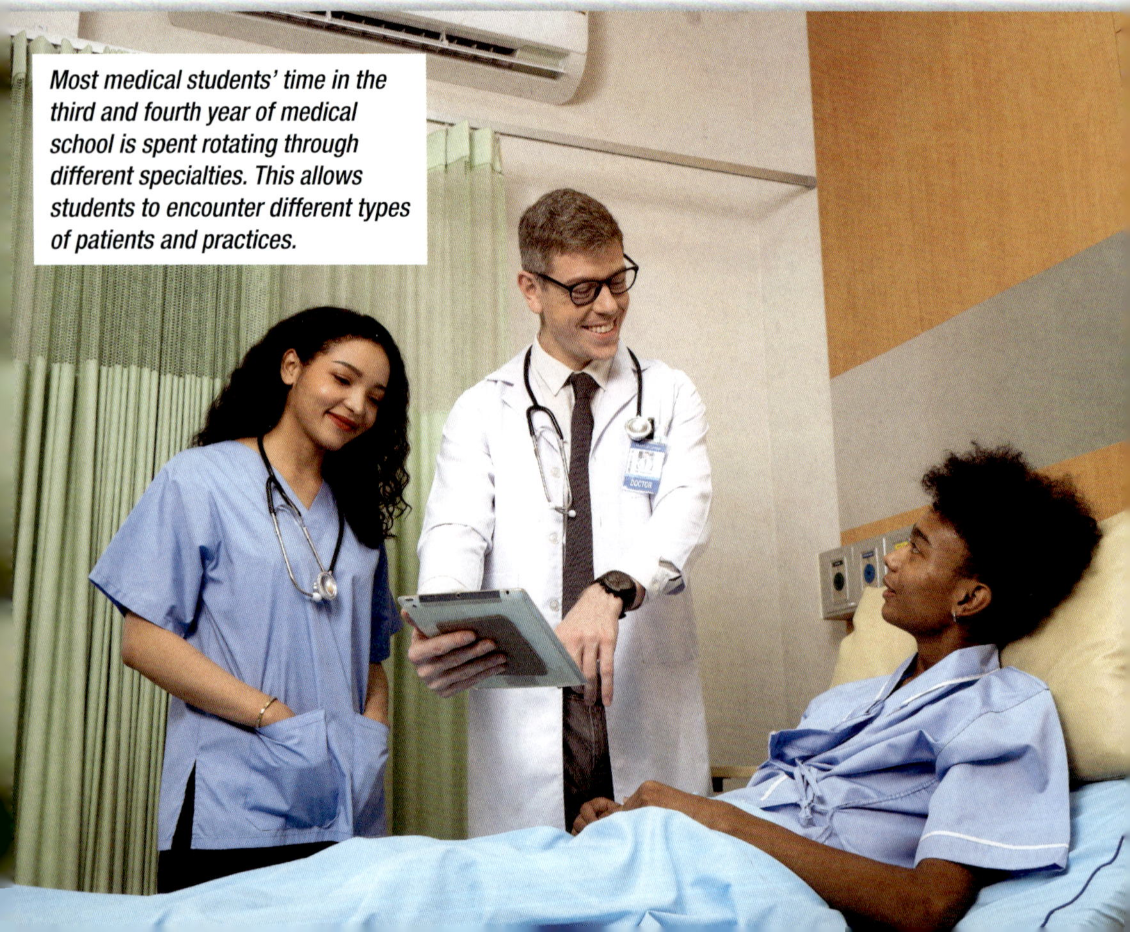

Most medical students' time in the third and fourth year of medical school is spent rotating through different specialties. This allows students to encounter different types of patients and practices.

During the third year of medical school, students have many of the same general rotations, including internal medicine, family medicine, OB-GYN, psychiatry, pediatrics, and emergency medicine. These give students the opportunity to acquire more foundational knowledge and encounter common ailments and conditions. Students have the opportunity to get hands-on experience examining patients, taking notes, and learning clinical skills while under the supervision of residents and attending doctors (often shortened to *attendings*). Throughout the years spent in clinical rotations, there are also opportunities to take a more active role in patient treatment. Maggie remembers her favorite parts of her surgery rotation, saying:

"The most exciting surgery days were when I spent the whole day in the OR and the residents were either out for lectures or the attending let the senior resident do the surgery on their own. In both scenarios, the medical student gets to be first assist and you get to do things that are way more fun than just holding an instrument and feeling like a 3rd wheel."[14]

—Maggie, medical student

> The most exciting surgery days were when I spent the whole day in the OR and the residents were either out for lectures or the attending let the senior resident do the surgery on their own. In both scenarios, the medical student gets to be first assist and you get to do things that are way more fun than just holding an instrument and feeling like a 3rd wheel. Some days I even got to do things like use the scalpel to put in port holes for laparoscopic surgeries, make the first incision on a spine surgery, and use the Bovie instrument as the surgeon told me where to cut.[14]

During the fourth year of medical school, students take on more elective rotations, as well as sub-internships, which allow them to audition at hospitals where they are interested in completing their residencies. Exploring the specialties and subspecialities they are interested during the third and fourth years can help students gain specialized experience, meet potential references, and decide what residencies to apply to.

CHAPTER THREE

Becoming a Doctor: Residency

While students graduating from medical school have received their DO or MD degree and are technically doctors, the process to become licensed and practice medicine independently takes several more years. The end of medical school is not the end of learning for these doctors. The residency process, which can last from three to seven years depending on the specialty chosen, is an opportunity for new doctors to acquire even more specialized knowledge and experience. They gain both by examining and treating patients under the supervision of more experienced doctors in clinic or hospital settings.

Applying for Residency

The process of applying for residency is an intense and demanding one, not unlike applying for medical school. Students must prepare an application that includes a personal statement, curriculum vitae (or résumé), transcripts, and recommendation letters. All of this must be submitted the summer before their last year of medical school. The most critical part of the process is interviews, which take place in the fall and winter. Students travel to the hospitals and clinics that grant them interviews. The interview process offers the opportunity for the programs to learn more about the applicants and the students to learn more about the programs. After the interview process is complete, students create a list of the programs they interviewed with in order of preference. This is officially known as a rank order list. The residency programs also create a list ranking their top candidates from the students they interviewed.

These lists are then used in the National Resident Matching Program to match medical students with residency positions. Students find out on the third Monday of March whether they have matched, but not with which program. This allows unmatched applicants to apply to any unfilled positions. Later that week, Match Day occurs. On this day residency matches are released to students by email and then are announced publicly in a ceremony at each medical school. "I felt as if I could not hear or see beyond my computer screen as my email was loading. I just remember reading the words 'Kresge Eye Institute' and starting to jump and dance," says Michael Saad of Wayne State University School of Medicine of the Match Day experience. "Once it finally hit me that I would be training at my top-ranked program, I felt excited for what's to come and proud to have come this far."[15] The National Resident Matching Program recorded 44,853 applicants submitting rank order lists, the highest ever, for 41,503 residency position openings in 2024.

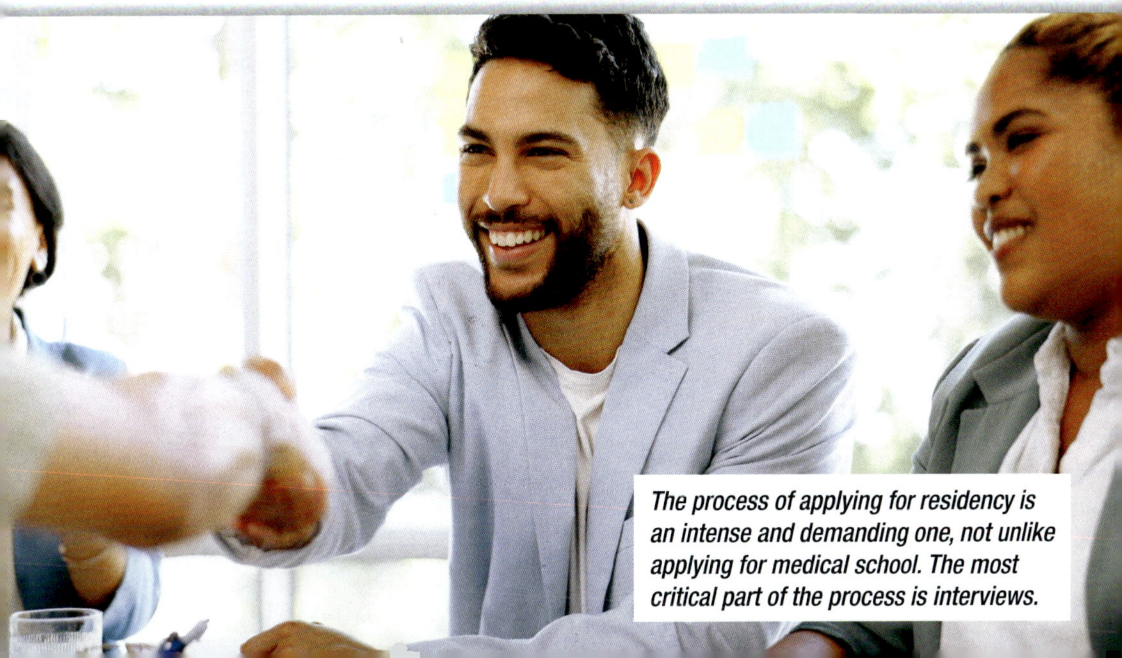

The process of applying for residency is an intense and demanding one, not unlike applying for medical school. The most critical part of the process is interviews.

What to Expect During Residency

If medical school sounds intense, residency is even more so. Students should prepare for some long hours during these years. The Accreditation Council for Graduate Medical Education restricts residents to working eighty hours a week. This is based on a four-week average, so some weeks residents may work more and some weeks less than eighty hours. Eight hours are required between scheduled shifts, and residents must have four days off over the course of four weeks. For most doctors, residency is the busiest and most challenging time in their career. In addition to working longer hours than attending doctors, residents' salaries are much lower than attendings'. Medscape's 2023 *Resident Salary and Debt Report* found that the average resident salary was $67,400. Among those surveyed, 76 percent expressed the view that this is unfair compensation.

While many residents have similar salaries and work hours, specialties chosen determine differences in what residents are doing on a daily basis and how long their residencies last. The short-

Fellowships for Further Specialization

After four years of medical school and three to seven years in residency, many doctors jump into beginning their careers as attending doctors. But some choose instead to complete a fellowship for further specialization. Fellowships add one to three years onto the educational experience of becoming a doctor. In 2024 the American Medical Association listed 130 fellowship subspecialties. These are some examples of opportunities for further specialization:

- In pediatrics: child abuse pediatrics, developmental-behavioral pediatrics, pediatric emergency medicine
- In psychiatry: addiction psychiatry, child and adolescent psychiatry, forensic psychiatry
- In surgery: hand surgery, vascular surgery, craniofacial surgery
- In OB-GYN: maternal-fetal medicine, complex family planning, female pelvic medicine and reconstructive surgery

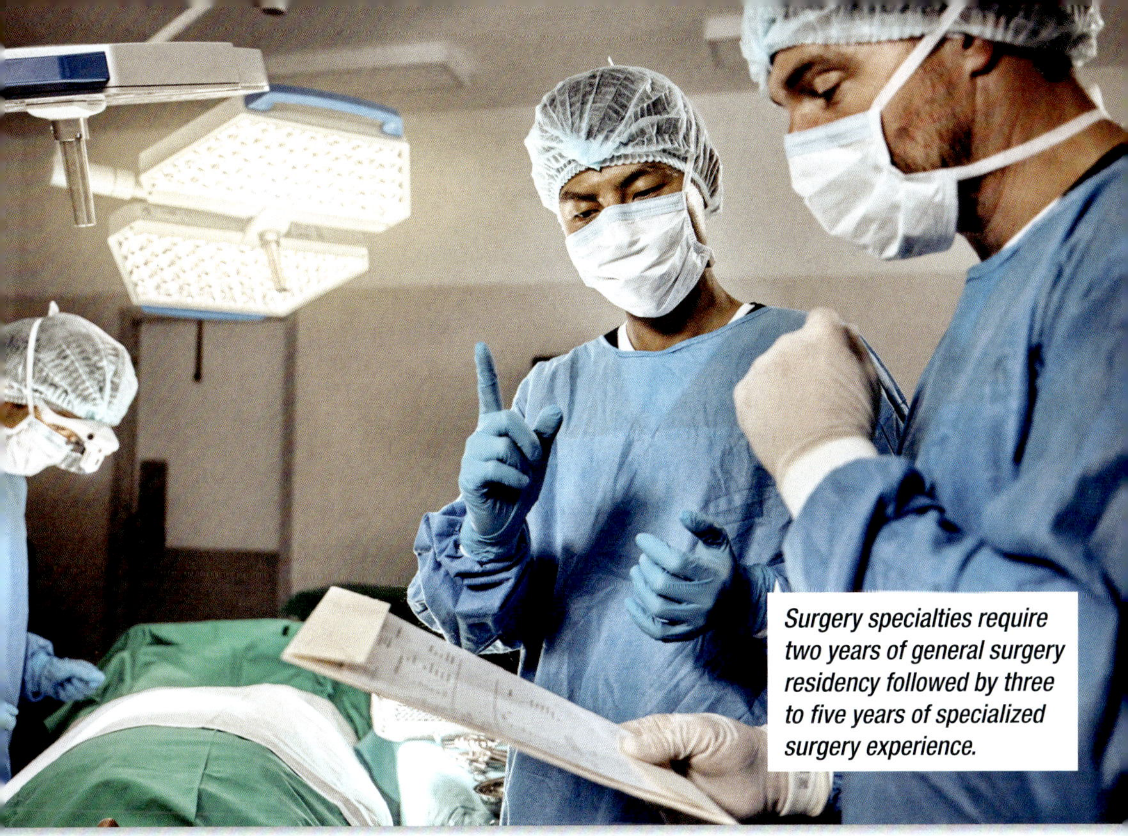

Surgery specialties require two years of general surgery residency followed by three to five years of specialized surgery experience.

est residencies at three to four years are generalist and primary care specialties, including emergency medicine, family medicine, internal medicine, pediatrics, and OB-GYN. The longest residencies at six to seven years include specialties like interventional radiology, neurological surgery, plastic surgery, and thoracic surgery. Surgery specialties require two years of general surgery residency followed by three to five years of specialized surgery experience.

The Intern Year

In the first year of residency, residents are known as interns. This is often considered the most challenging year of residency, as interns adjust to the long hours and the responsibility of more direct patient care. During this year, interns' care of patients is supervised by chief residents and attending doctors, and they rotate through different subspecialties. Along with seeing patients, residents in all years attend lectures and participate in skills labs, where they collectively discuss challenging patient cases. A typical shift begins with receiving updates from the doctors on the

> "8:15–11:00 am [is] rounds with the whole team. We typically start with new or unstable patients. This is when we perform our formal presentations and discuss differential diagnoses and plans for our patients. Applicable bedside teaching happens here as well!"[16]
>
> —Dr. Annie Kopera, internal medicine intern

previous shift and then conducting pre-rounds and rounds, which involve visiting assigned patients individually and as a group of residents. Interns might check lab work and patient vitals (such as temperature and pulse rate), do physical examinations, and gather medical histories for new patients. Dr. Annie Kopera describes this part of her day, beginning with pre-rounds and then moving on to rounds, as an internal medicine intern:

> I will see how all my existing patients did overnight, and get a more thorough story from my new patients. I like to check in with the nursing staff quickly to see if they have any specific concerns for any patients. 8:15–11:00 am [is] rounds with the whole team. We typically start with new or unstable patients. This is when we perform our formal presentations and discuss differential diagnoses and plans for our patients. Applicable bedside teaching happens here as well![16]

Another key part of the intern experience is learning the ins and outs of charting, which is keeping the records on individual patients. A patient's chart is the record of everything that is ordered (all lab tests, procedures, scans, and so on), encounters with staff, and the treatment plan for the patient's stay in the hospital. Residents can spend up to 42 percent of their day charting, which is often more than time spent directly with patients. An intern's day also might include communicating with patients' families and other members of their medical care team.

The intern year is not all about medical records and exams though. Interns often are called in for more hands-on experience treating patients. An intern at Henry Ford Macomb Hospital recalls this experience with a code blue, which is a patient medical emergency such as someone's heart stopping. The intern describes the

Work-Life Balance During Residency

One of the biggest challenges during residency is the workload. It is important for residents to be intentional about managing stress, establishing boundaries between work and home life, and keeping their bodies and minds healthy to avoid burnout. Here are some things that are important for residents to keep in mind:

- **Take care of your body.** Eating healthy and finding time for exercise, even if it's just a walk during a break or at shift's end, is key to keeping yourself well and reducing stress. It can be easy to skip meals or ignore what your body is telling you it needs when you are focusing on the needs of others all day.
- **Find someone to vent to.** Whether it is a friend, a therapist, or your fellow residents, you will need an outlet to process stress and complicated feelings that might result from you encountering death and upsetting injuries and diagnoses.
- **Spend time each week doing something you love.** This could be spending time with friends and family, partaking in a favorite hobby, or spending time outdoors for a few hours—anything that can help you recharge.

experience, saying, "I get in line to do chest compressions. I observe the sequence of events: chest compressions, pulse check, Epi [epinephrine administered to try to restart the heart], etc, trying to retain it all. . . . I spend two minutes doing chest compressions, which feels like ten minutes with my weak arms. The patient eventually achieves ROSC [return of spontaneous circulation]!"[17]

Year Two and On

After year one of residency, doctors are officially known as residents. During the remainder of their residency, residents are still under the supervision of attending doctors, but they do have the opportunity to participate in more procedures and even surgeries while an attending is present. Clarence Cabatu, a second-year orthopedic surgery resident, explains some of his responsibilities: "Our responsibilities in the OR are to help prepare and drape the patient in [the] operating room, assist the attending surgeon

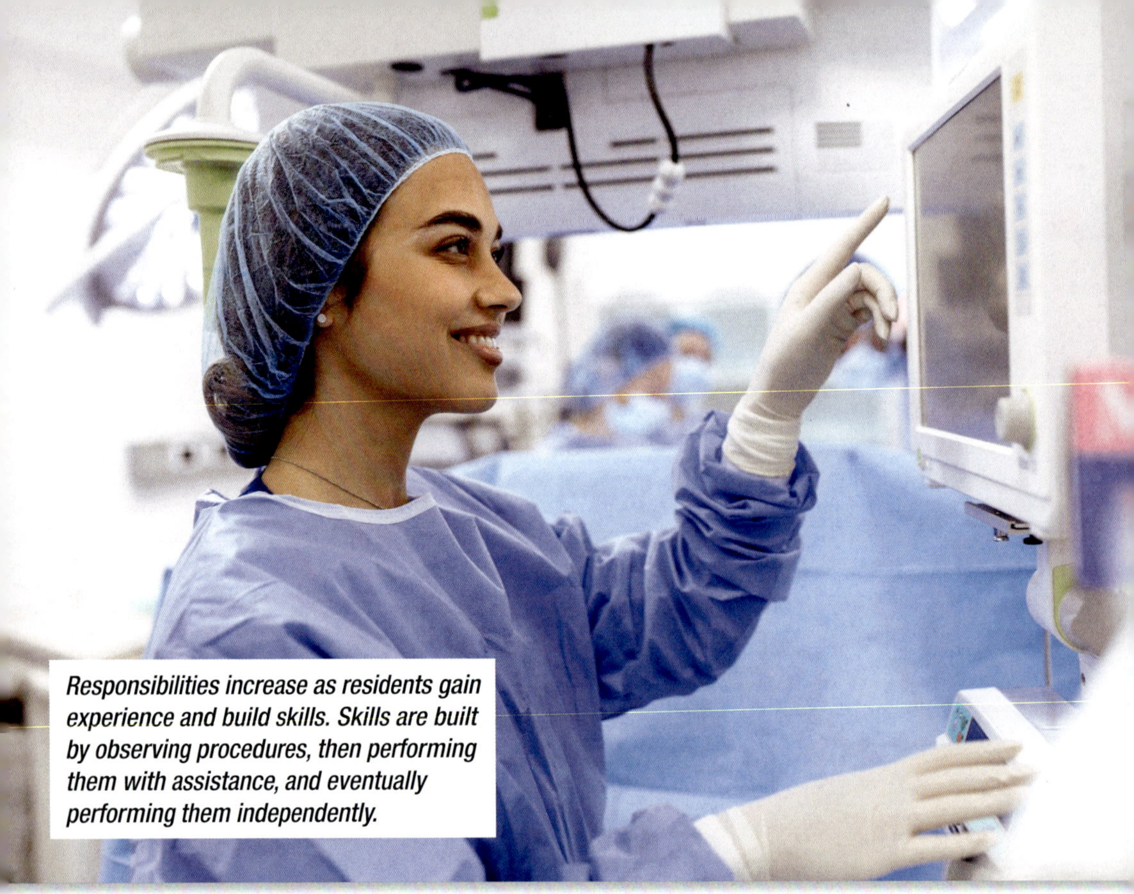

Responsibilities increase as residents gain experience and build skills. Skills are built by observing procedures, then performing them with assistance, and eventually performing them independently.

with the case, write post operative orders, and follow the patient's post op course. . . . Once a month, we have a simulation lab to practice our surgical skills on cadaveric models."[18]

Responsibilities increase each year of residency as residents gain experience and build skills. As in many other fields, skills are built by observing procedures, then performing them with assistance, and eventually performing them independently under supervision. Residents also have the opportunity to explore areas of interest that are in line with their future professional goals. Kavin Fatehchand, a fourth-year resident at Columbia University's Department of Psychiatry, says:

> I picked electives based on my own unique interests and professional goals. The majority of my year will be dedicated to continuing to provide longitudinal care to my patients in the Psychiatric Institute Resident Clinic, our outpatient

resident clinic and in OnTrack, Columbia's first break psychosis treatment program. As a queer trainee, I am also very interested in working with the queer population and will also be devoting time this year to co-leading a therapy group with non-binary/trans folks.[19]

Doctors who have completed medical school, done at least one year of residency, and passed the three-part medical licensing exam will apply to become a licensed doctor. Each state has its own individual requirements for medical licensing, and doctors have to renew their license regularly, usually every two years. Doctors also have the option to obtain board certification in their specialty and/or subspeciality. This includes further written and oral exams and is an expensive process, so not all doctors choose to become board certified. However, more hospitals are requiring board certification for doctors to practice medicine, and some health insurance companies will offer different levels of reimbursement based on whether a doctor is board certified, so it is becoming more of a necessity. Board certification proves that doctors have expertise in their area of specialty to both potential employers and patients seeking out specialists.

"Our responsibilities in the OR are to help prepare and drape the patient in [the] operating room, assist the attending surgeon with the case, write post operative orders, and follow the patient's post op course. . . . Once a month, we have a simulation lab to practice our surgical skills on cadaveric models."[18]

—Clarence Cabatu, second-year orthopedic surgery resident

CHAPTER FOUR

The Day-to-Day Work of a Doctor

The day-to-day work of a doctor can vary due to both the setting and specialty chosen. Most doctors work either in a hospital, clinic, or private-practice doctor's office. In a hospital setting, doctors typically have fewer administrative tasks and more time to focus on clinical activities. They also usually have a set salary. Doctors who have their own private practice or who work with a private-practice group have the independence of being their own boss, with the added workload of also running a business. Doctors who are employed at private practices also like being able to form relationships with patients they see regularly. According to Medscape's physician compensation report, doctors in private practice average $52,000 more in pay per year. However, the differences in their workdays are mostly affected by the specialty they practice.

The following are typical days of pediatricians, psychiatrists, ER doctors, and cardiac surgeons. The descriptions include insights from real doctors currently practicing those specialties.

Pediatricians

Many primary care pediatricians typically begin their day by checking their email or internal messaging system and voicemail for messages that need to be addressed immediately. They might see prescription refill requests, which they will send into patients' pharmacies. Or they might see messages from parents concerned with their child's diaper rash or fever. In situations like this, pediatricians might message the parents asking them to set up telehealth or in-person appointments for later that day.

Pediatricians see children (and their parents) when children are sick or when a problem arises. For instance, pediatricians might hear from the concerned parents of a week-old infant who is not producing enough wet diapers and seems to be losing weight. The pediatrician might suggest that the breastfeeding mother supplement with formula and schedule an appointment for the next day for the baby to be weighed again. The doctor might have a telehealth visit for the toddler with diaper rash. After viewing the rash on camera, the doctor might suggest medicated cream and cleaning with water and cotton pads instead of wipes until the rash heals. Between appointments, it is not uncommon for pediatricians to once again check and respond to more messages from parents. Other sick visits could include a six-year-old with an ear infection who is prescribed antibiotics and a preteen who is struggling with anxiety and refusing to go to school.

Most days pediatricians also perform well checks on their young patients. These are routine physical exams during which

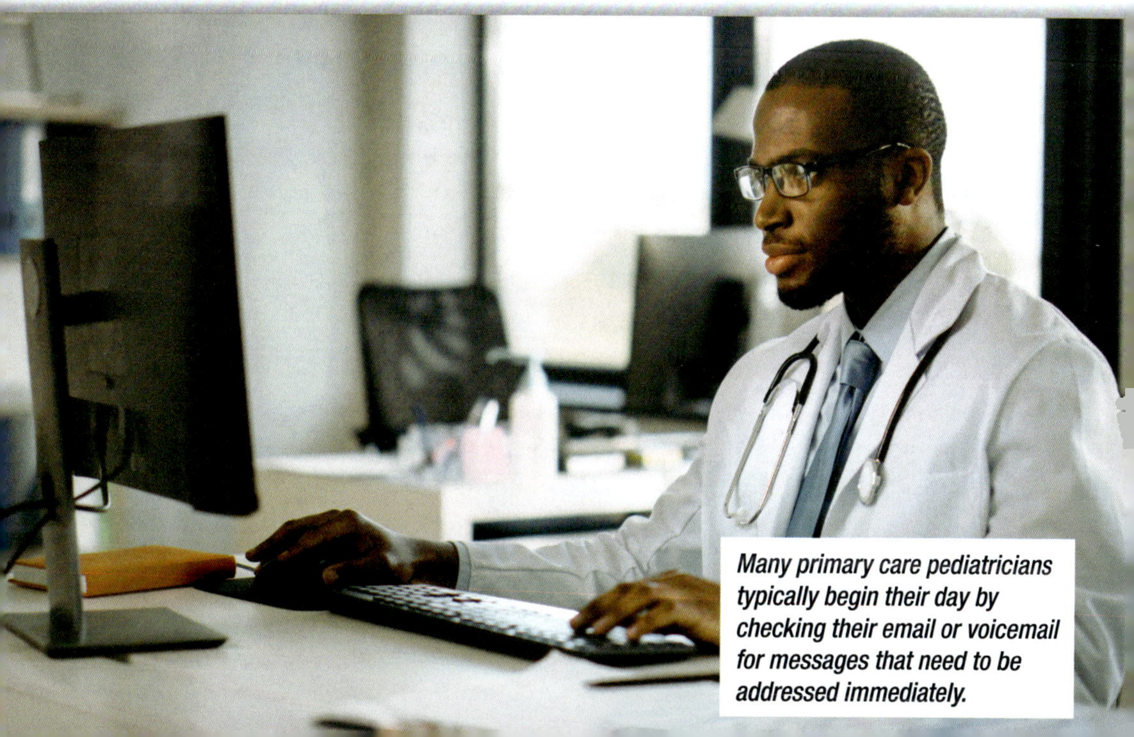

Many primary care pediatricians typically begin their day by checking their email or voicemail for messages that need to be addressed immediately.

pediatricians check on growth and developmental progress. They also use these visits to provide age-appropriate information to parents and answer questions. Dr. Rei Tosu, a pediatrician at Los Alamitos Pediatrics in California, describes a six-month well check with one of her patients:

> Mom tells me that he has started eating solids and I can see during his exam that he is now sitting well on his own. He seems to be growing and developing well! I talk to the mom about child-proofing the home, since the chances are good that this little boy will be mobile before his next visit. During this visit, he receives his 6-month vaccines plus the flu vaccine. I'm looking forward to seeing this baby again during his next well-check. He will have grown so much![20]

"Kids don't vote, they have no lobby, they don't get to pick what they have for dinner—they have no say. And sometimes the people responsible for them don't make the best choices for them. But as a pediatrician, you have the opportunity to advocate for them! If you can do that, because they're so little, you can have such a huge impact on their lives."[21]

—Emanuele M., pediatrician

During a well visit, a pediatrician might observe developmental concerns. When combined with a parent's answers to the developmental questionnaire, for instance, the doctor might recommend pursuing autism screening or seeking intervention for a child who is not meeting milestones for gross or fine motor skills. The doctor will also provide the parents with a list of providers in the area to call. Pediatrician Emanuele M. says that the difference he can make in children's lives is the best part of being a pediatrician. "Kids don't vote, they have no lobby, they don't get to pick what they have for dinner—they have no say. And sometimes the people responsible for them don't make the best choices for them," he says, "But as a pediatrician, you have the opportunity to advocate for them! If you can do that, because they're so little, you can have such a huge impact on their lives."[21]

Part of a Pediatrician's Day

"1 p.m.—I take the opportunity to prep the charts for the following day. I . . . notice I have a 3-year-old new patient. I go into her chart and notice she has had multiple specialist visits. I spend some time reading to find out she was diagnosed with kidney cancer and has been under treatment but is now in remission. One of the advantages of being part of . . . [a] Primary Care Network is that the electronic medical record platform is the same for all . . . providers and I am able to access notes from her . . . specialists and studies that have been done. Even though I will be meeting this patient for the first time tomorrow, I already feel well-versed with her medical history and feel comfortable taking care of her.

1:30 p.m.—I get ready for another telehealth appointment on Zoom, this time with a pregnant mom for her prenatal consult. She is expecting a baby boy next month, and I answer some questions she has about newborn care and circumcision. It's nice for both sides to put faces to names before we meet for the first time when the baby is delivered."

—Dr. Rei Tosu, pediatrician at Los Alamitos Pediatrics in California

Rei Tosu, "A Day in the Life of a Pediatrician," CHOC Inside, March 22, 2022. https://inside.choc.org.

Emergency Medicine Doctors

The specialty of emergency medicine is one of the fastest paced in the field and also involves encountering a wide variety of cases. Dr. Kathleen Clem went into emergency medicine for exactly that reason. "The entire shift is going to be a mystery until I get into it. And not knowing what's coming through the door is part of the fun of what I do," she says, "To go through an emergency with someone, to be qualified and trained to help them and make the emergency turn out as well as possible—really is what keeps me going."[22] For ER doctors like Clem, shifts vary from eight to twelve hours, and they have three to five a week, adding up to about forty hours. There are patients waiting to be seen, as well as ambulances with trauma patients arriving regularly.

ER doctors might encounter a four-year-old child who has fallen from a piece of playground equipment and has a suspected broken arm. They will conduct a physical examination and order an X-ray for the arm. If the X-rays show that the child does have a

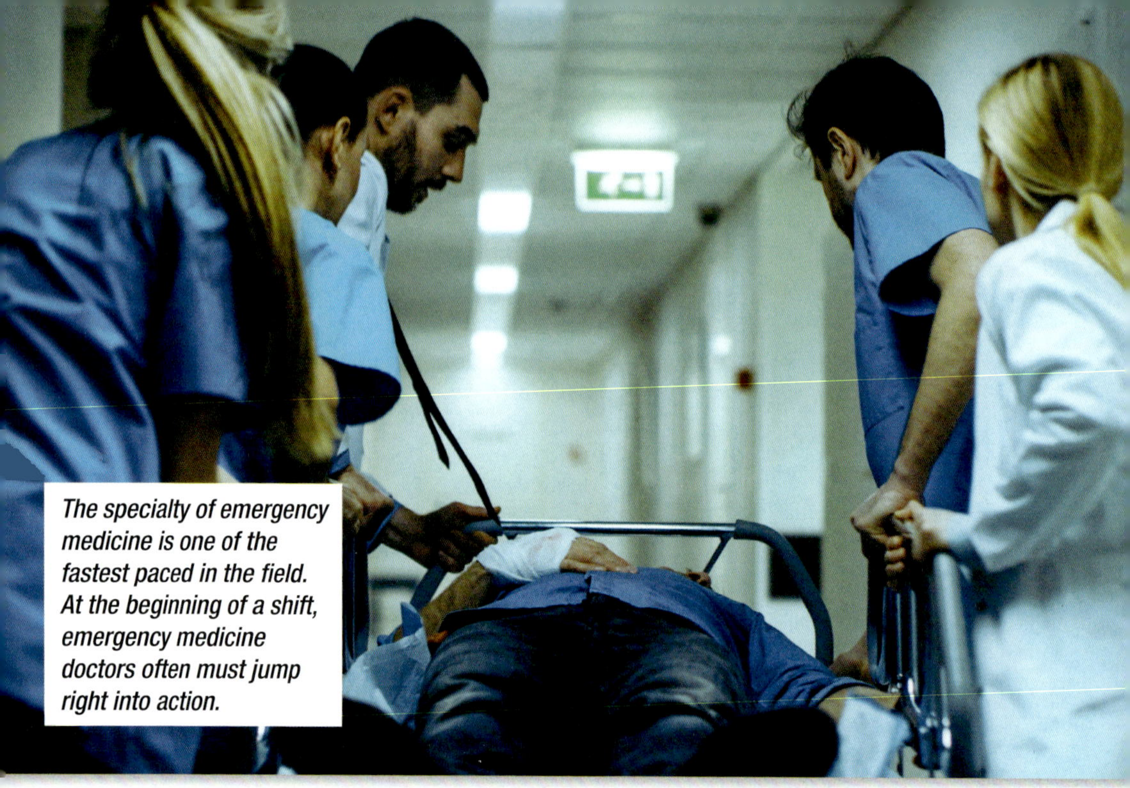

The specialty of emergency medicine is one of the fastest paced in the field. At the beginning of a shift, emergency medicine doctors often must jump right into action.

broken arm, an ER doctor will set and cast the arm while the child is under sedation.

Visits with stable patients might be interrupted by incoming trauma cases, such as a pedestrian hit by a car. In the emergency room a triage approach is used, which means that a staff member, often a triage nurse, determines the most urgent needs to be seen first. A trauma case could involve multiple lacerations, broken bones, and possible internal bleeding. The doctor will conduct a quick examination and then address the most urgent needs—including stopping bleeding—as monitoring equipment is attached, oxygen is provided, and veins are accessed for intravenous lines by other staff members. A call might be made to the surgery department and the patient sent to the OR if surgery is needed to further address injuries. An ER doctor also might encounter patients experiencing symptoms of a heart attack. If the patient goes into cardiac arrest, the ER team will attempt resuscitation. ER doctors often consult with specialists, such as the on-call cardiologist in the case of a heart attack. The patient might be admitted to the hospital for a full cardiac assessment and testing.

Sometimes patients visit the ER for symptoms or conditions that are not critical, but there are many times that ER doctors encounter severe trauma, disappointing outcomes, and even deaths. Dr. Val Vigil, an ER doctor at Natividad Hospital in California, describes her experience of one of these cases:

> I see paramedics and firefighters rushing in a young man on a breathing mask. I have a horrible feeling when I realize it's a young man with a drug overdose who was just discharged only hours ago—even after extensive counseling about drug use. . . . By the report, he went home and must have taken additional fentanyl/oxy (oxycodone) and possibly other drugs such as Xanax—and was found down on the floor, hardly breathing. This time he looks worse than last time. This time he will need a breathing tube and may not recover.[23]

Psychiatrists

"I see paramedics and firefighters rushing in a young man on a breathing mask. I have a horrible feeling when I realize it's a young man with a drug overdose who was just discharged only hours ago—even after extensive counseling about drug use. . . . This time he looks worse than last time. This time he will need a breathing tube and may not recover."[23]

—Val Vigil, ER doctor

Most psychiatrists start their days by reviewing any messages from patients. These messages will be returned, medication refill requests will be approved, and communication with other members of patients' treatment teams will take place. Psychiatrists are trained to offer psychotherapy and also, as MDs, are licensed to prescribe medications, unlike psychologists or counselors. Some do both, but many psychiatrists offer only the service of medication management. Psychiatrists will see patients regularly for medication management appointments. A patient might be experiencing higher stress and some seasonal changes in his or her depression, so a change in dosage of the patient's prescribed antidepressant could be called into the pharmacy. If psychiatrists have space in their schedules for new patients, they will also have introductory appointments. Psychiatrists will take a history of each patient's mental health, record medications tried in the past, and ask a lot of questions to decide which new medication regime might be best for each individual patient. Regular follow-up appointments are made to assess how each patient is reacting to any changes in medication or in their mental health.

Being a psychiatrist can often be mentally and emotionally draining. With mental illness, unfortunate outcomes can occur, and it also can be difficult to see patients suffering when there is no easy fix available. Dr. Shailesh Jain, a child and adolescent psychiatrist, describes a teenager under her care who decided to enter an inpatient psychiatric unit after initially trying to avoid it. "He has been struggling with intense anxiety and depression but has been resisting admission. We have been meeting almost every other day for the past two weeks and engaging in intense

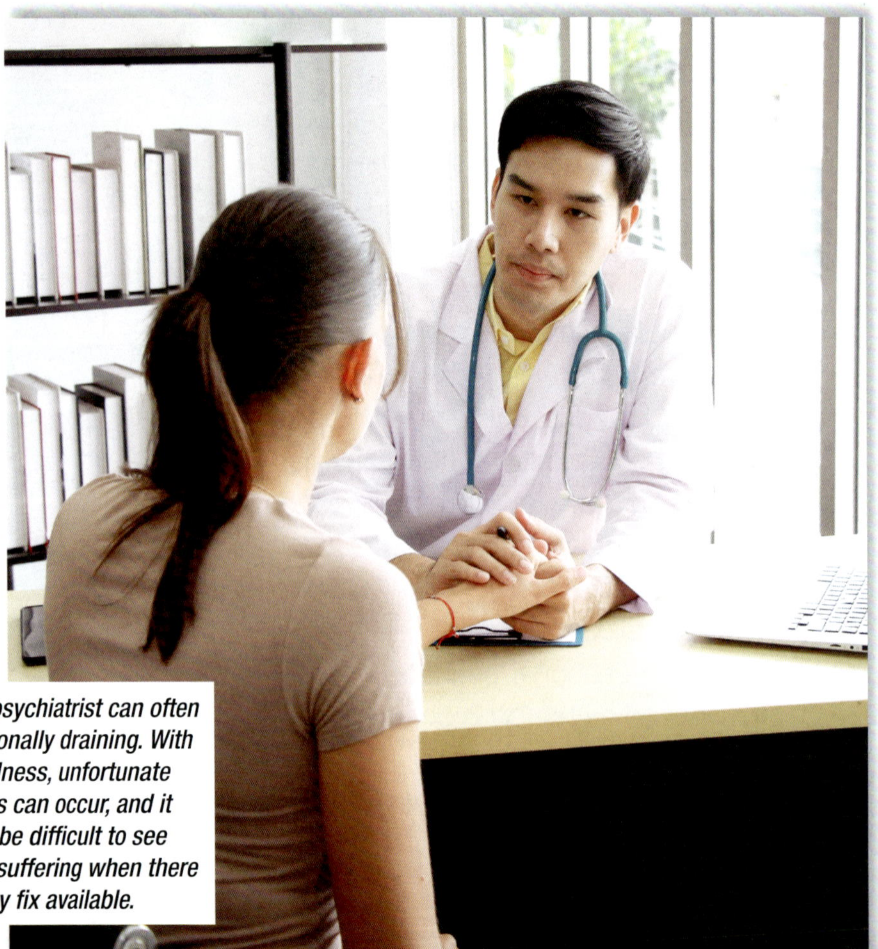

Being a psychiatrist can often be emotionally draining. With mental illness, unfortunate outcomes can occur, and it also can be difficult to see patients suffering when there is no easy fix available.

The Challenges of ER Medicine

"The hardest thing for me is patients with unrealistic expectations. In certain instances, patients think that 'No matter what's wrong with me I'm going to the ER and that doctor should figure it out and provide a cure,' or 'I have this problem I have had for a long time and I'm going to go the ER and my problem is going to be fixed right away.'

Those kinds of things are difficult. It's also difficult when a patient comes in with the expectation they will be admitted to the hospital, and it turns out that it's safe for them to have their work-ups done—after we check for an emergency—as an outpatient. They can be very disappointed and feel that the emergency physician should have the power to admit them. . . .

It is also difficult to find outpatient mental health care. We know what the patient needs, but we can't find the resources outside the emergency department. I cope with this by reminding myself that at least they can see me in the emergency department today."

—Dr. Kathleen Clem, emergency medicine provider

Kathleen Clem, "What It's like to Specialize in Emergency Medicine: Shadowing Dr. Clem," American Medical Association, January 26, 2024. www.ama-assn.org.

cognitive therapy to assess his core issues and distortions in his thinking. Should his condition deteriorate, he has access to my cell number and email. It has been emotionally draining for me."[24]

Cardiac Surgeons

Similar to ER doctors, cardiac surgeons can face days that are both demanding and unpredictable. Part of a typical workweek is spent on surgeries, but cardiac surgeons also spend time monitoring patients in intensive care, doing rounds, and conducting research. Since emergency surgeries may come in, surgeons also have assigned on-call times when they aren't on shift but remain ready to return to the hospital as needed. Cardiac surgeons spend part of their shifts visiting patients in the intensive care unit to monitor their progress and determine whether they can be moved into the recovery part of the hospital. Open heart surgery often requires five to seven days of recovery in the hospital.

A fairly common surgery conducted by cardiac surgeons is a coronary artery bypass graft, which takes three to six hours. A surgeon will first remove the blood vessels being used (usually from the arms or legs) and then graft them onto the aorta to bypass diseased or blocked vessels. Dr. Alexander Marmureanu says of this common procedure, "I have done a hundred last year. None of them are the same. Every single one is different. It's like driving from your home to your office and every day taking a different route, different weather, different car, different street, or a different scenario. That's the same thing with those operations."[25] After surgeons have completed surgeries, they usually update any waiting family members.

Annuloplasty valve repair, which involves sewing a band around the ring of a heart valve to reinforce and tighten the existing valve and improve blood flow, is another common surgery for a cardiac surgeon. Dr. Paul Massimiano, a cardiac and thoracic surgeon at Adventist HealthCare White Oak Medical Center, says the environment for an operation like this "is like a well choreographed ballet. Everyone knows their role. The technicians, and the scrub techs, and the perfusionists who run the heart lung machine, all these people are very sophisticated. They all know exactly what to do. So the environment is very controlled."[26]

Different Specialties, Different Lives

Medical students' personalities, types of patients they desire to work with, scientific interests, and ability to handle stress and high-pressure situations should all be taken into consideration when determining what kind of medicine they want to pursue as a career. Some may prefer the ability to build relationships as a pediatrician and watch children grow up, while the fast-paced, adrenaline-filled life of an ER doctor may be the right fit for another person.

CHAPTER FIVE

What Skills and Personal Qualities Are Needed?

Being a doctor is a demanding job, physically, mentally, and emotionally. Staying the course through the challenges of training and then practicing medicine requires stamina and persistence, along with other critical skills and personal qualities. Some of these qualities may be ones that doctors had prior to entering medical school, but others can be learned or enhanced during the medical school and residency process. Intelligence, the ability to retain large amounts of information, and curiosity are key to being successful first in medical school and eventually as a licensed doctor serving patients with many different needs. Doctors who work closely with patients also need to be able to express empathy and compassion and effectively communicate. It is also important for doctors to be both confident and humble and able to collaborate with their colleagues.

Persistence

Persistence and commitment are critical to making it through the four years of medical school and three to seven years of residency required to be a doctor. Students who are interested in working as a doctor have to really want it and must have the tenacity to make it through those years. Ross University School of Medicine notes that resilience is a part of this: "A medical career comes with its share of hardships, and resilience is important for any doctor's long-term success. Long hours, hard work, and stress can lead to burnout, a condition of emotional and physical exhaustion. Physicians must be able to bounce back from burnout, as well as when they face emotionally difficult circumstances."[27] This persistence will also help when pursuing diagnoses and advocating for patients throughout their careers.

Intelligence and Curiosity

It may seem like a no-brainer that doctors must be smart, but this goes deeper than just being able to absorb and remember lots of complex information. Dr. Kevin Jubbal of Med School Insiders says that during medical school, "if you're incredibly brilliant but don't know how to study effectively, you will not succeed. . . . While a strong intellect certainly helps, what matters most is developing a rock-solid work ethic, healthy habits, and effective study strategies you can stick to."[28] These learned study skills can also be applied to being detail oriented and organized throughout a doctor's career, which is key for accurate record keeping and making sure patients get the correct tests and aftercare instructions.

> "If you're incredibly brilliant but don't know how to study effectively, you will not succeed. . . . While a strong intellect certainly helps, what matters most is developing a rock-solid work ethic, healthy habits, and effective study strategies you can stick to."[28]
>
> —Dr. Kevin Jubbal, Med School Insiders

Doctors also must have the intelligence to apply what they have learned to individual patients. A sense of curiosity and interest in problem solving is important, because good doctors continue to learn about new developments in the medical field and seek out new treatment options for their patients. When doctors encounter patients with unusual or difficult-to-diagnose symptoms, they have to be willing to follow the symptoms almost like a detective.

Confidence and Humility

Confidence and humility are both qualities that are important for doctors to have. Confidence is not the same as cockiness or believ-

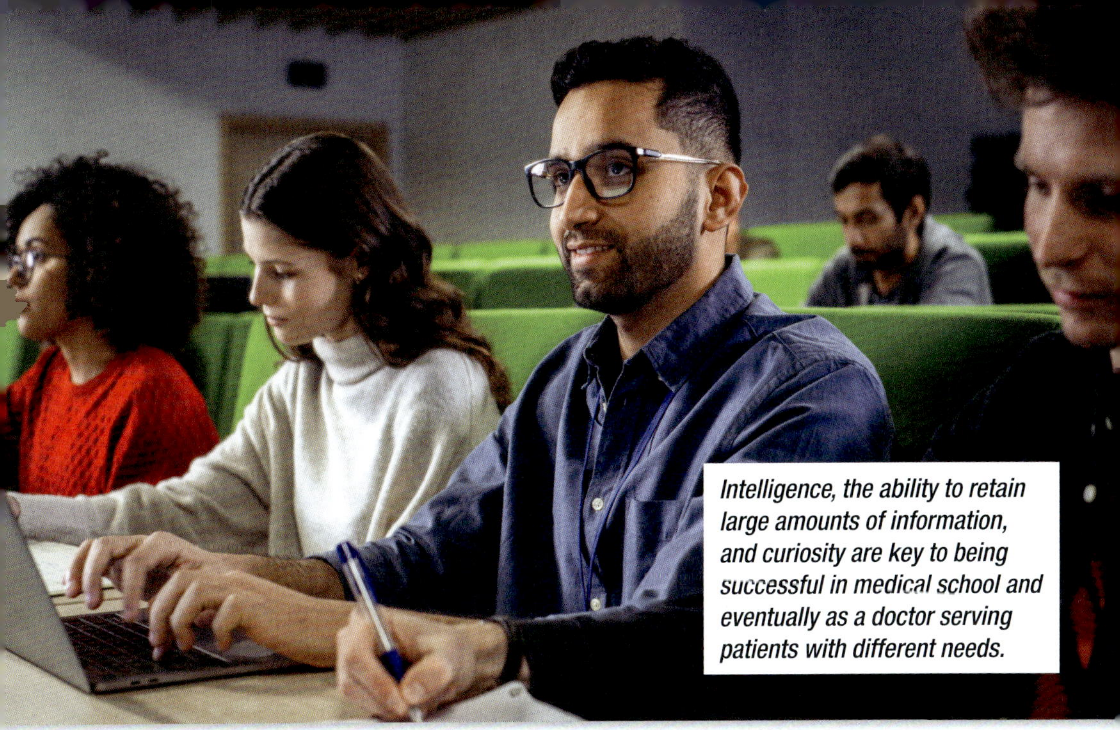

Intelligence, the ability to retain large amounts of information, and curiosity are key to being successful in medical school and eventually as a doctor serving patients with different needs.

ing that you are better or smarter than other people. It is important that doctors are confident in both their abilities as a doctor and their diagnoses and treatments for patients; otherwise, they will be unable to do their job effectively or even at all. Humility is necessary to be able to work in a collaborative setting and not let pride get in the way of digging deeper for diagnoses that might not be obvious.

Dr. Ami DeWaters, an associate professor of medicine at Penn State College of Medicine, says:

> Some would argue that humility is a personal characteristic you either have or don't. I wouldn't agree with that, necessarily. You can learn how to question yourself and approach a situation in a more intellectually humble manner by doing things like asking, "How would a colleague in a different field approach this case? What assumptions am I making that I should challenge right now?"[29]

Humility also reminds doctors to always keep learning and to explain medical diagnoses and aftercare to patients in a way that they can understand.

Good Bedside Manner

Bedside manner can be summed up as a doctor's people skills. While there are many doctors who have not mastered good bedside manner, it is critical to being a good doctor. It encompasses having patience, compassion, and good listening and communication skills. The ability to be an active listener and communicate complicated medical information in an understandable way to patients can be key to obtaining accurate diagnoses and making sure patients are able to carry out instructions for treatment. Patients are also more likely to open up with and feel well cared for by doctors who express empathy and kindness during visits. Dr. Joseph S. Alpert of the University of Arizona Department of Medicine says:

> The most important feature of a good doctor [is] kindness closely allied with empathy. . . . Sheer knowledge alone without a hefty dose of kindness and empathy, major elements of our humanity, will mean that the "kindness- and empathy-deficient" doctor will not be able to understand what the patient is experiencing and will also not be able to forge a strong and caring relationship with that patient.[30]

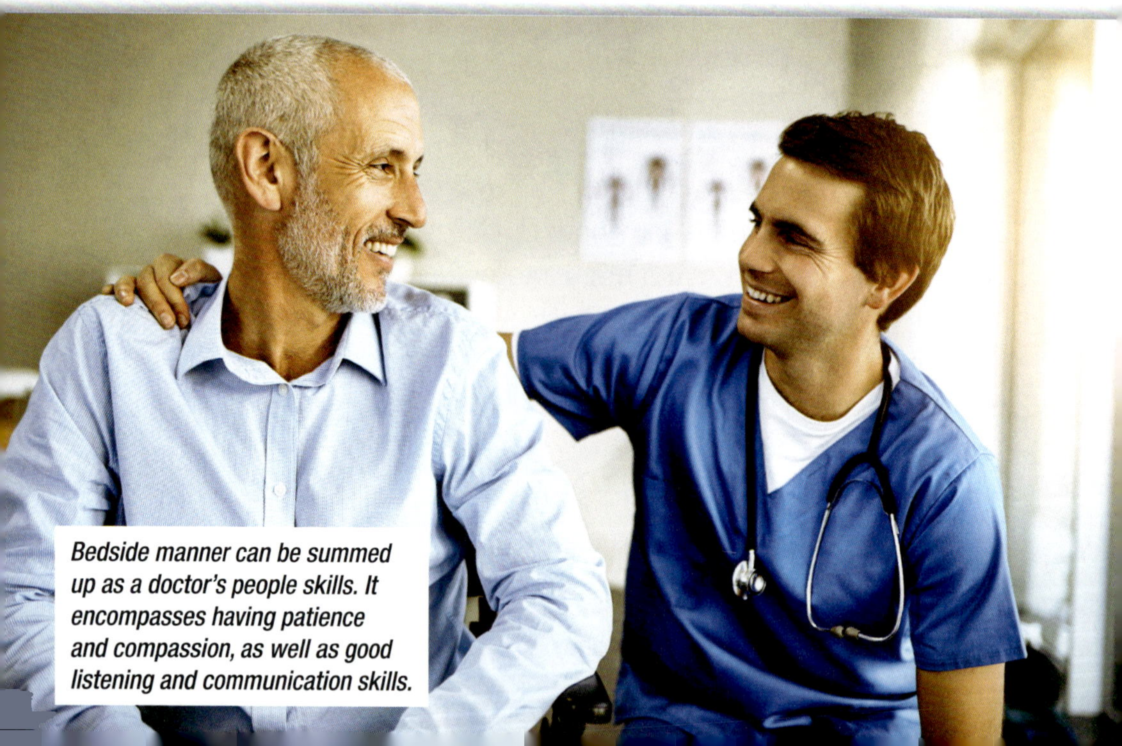

Bedside manner can be summed up as a doctor's people skills. It encompasses having patience and compassion, as well as good listening and communication skills.

What Do Patients Most Want from Their Doctors?

The *U.S. News & World Report*'s 2024 Primary Care Experience Survey found that only 73 percent of those surveyed had an annual physical in 2023 or 2024. While some don't schedule visits due to scheduling conflicts or financial worries, many avoid visiting the doctor due to having had poor experiences previously. Twenty-five percent reported they didn't go because they didn't like going to the doctor, and 10 percent had felt judged by doctors in the past. Here are some of the qualities survey participants said are most important for their doctors to have:

- Trustworthiness
- Compassion and empathy
- Ability to make them feel comfortable
- Open communication
- Ability to help them feel heard and understood
- Ability to be nonjudgmental
- Ability to explain things well

Learning to Be a Doctor

While medical school and residency are primarily filled with learning scientific knowledge, observing and practicing the skills and qualities needed to become a good doctor also are an important part of the learning experience. Many doctors believe that qualities such as humility, empathy, and good communication skills can be learned throughout this process. Armed with persistence, curiosity, and a desire for learning and growth, current medical school students and residents are able to develop into the empathic problem solvers we need as the doctors of the future.

"Sheer knowledge alone without a hefty dose of kindness and empathy, major elements of our humanity, will mean that the 'kindness- and empathy-deficient' doctor will not be able to understand what the patient is experiencing and will also not be able to forge a strong and caring relationship with that patient."[30]

—Dr. Joseph S. Alpert, University of Arizona Department of Medicine

CHAPTER SIX

Looking to the Future

The demand for doctors and for other jobs in the medical field continues to grow. This is unlikely to change since we as humans continue to have a need for medical treatment. Innovations in medicine, including medical research and advances in technology, have not decreased this demand. Rather, they have given doctors new forms of treatment and opportunities to treat patients who might have been untreatable or had no access to treatment in the past. These changes in the medical field also give doctors the opportunity to explore other career avenues that utilize their degrees and training, such as jobs in medical research and medical technology.

The Demand for Doctors

Doctors retiring and leaving the field for other reasons means that there is a consistent need for new doctors to take their place, especially in primary care specialties such as family medicine and psychiatry. The increase in the number of chronically ill Americans also has had an impact on this demand. The Bureau of Labor Statistics projects 3 percent growth in jobs for doctors, or about 24,200 new doctors needed each year through 2032 to keep up with demand. There is 4 percent projected growth for family medicine doctors, 7 percent for psychiatrists, and 5 percent for pathologists. In the 2022–2023 school year, there were 20,920 medical school graduates from US medical schools—a number that is shy of the projected need.

Alternate Jobs for Doctors

Some doctors will choose to practice clinical medicine for the entirety of their career. Others will decide to pivot away from patient care into jobs that still make use of their medical degrees and years of clinical experience. According to the *New England Journal of Medicine* CareerCenter, this transition is much easier than it was in the past. There are many reasons that a doctor might explore other jobs, says the center, but "the key ones are a desire to seek new challenges or the awakening that full-time patient care isn't the best fit. In some cases, physicians pursue nonclinical work almost by happenstance, when they're exposed to something in the course of their clinical practice."[31]

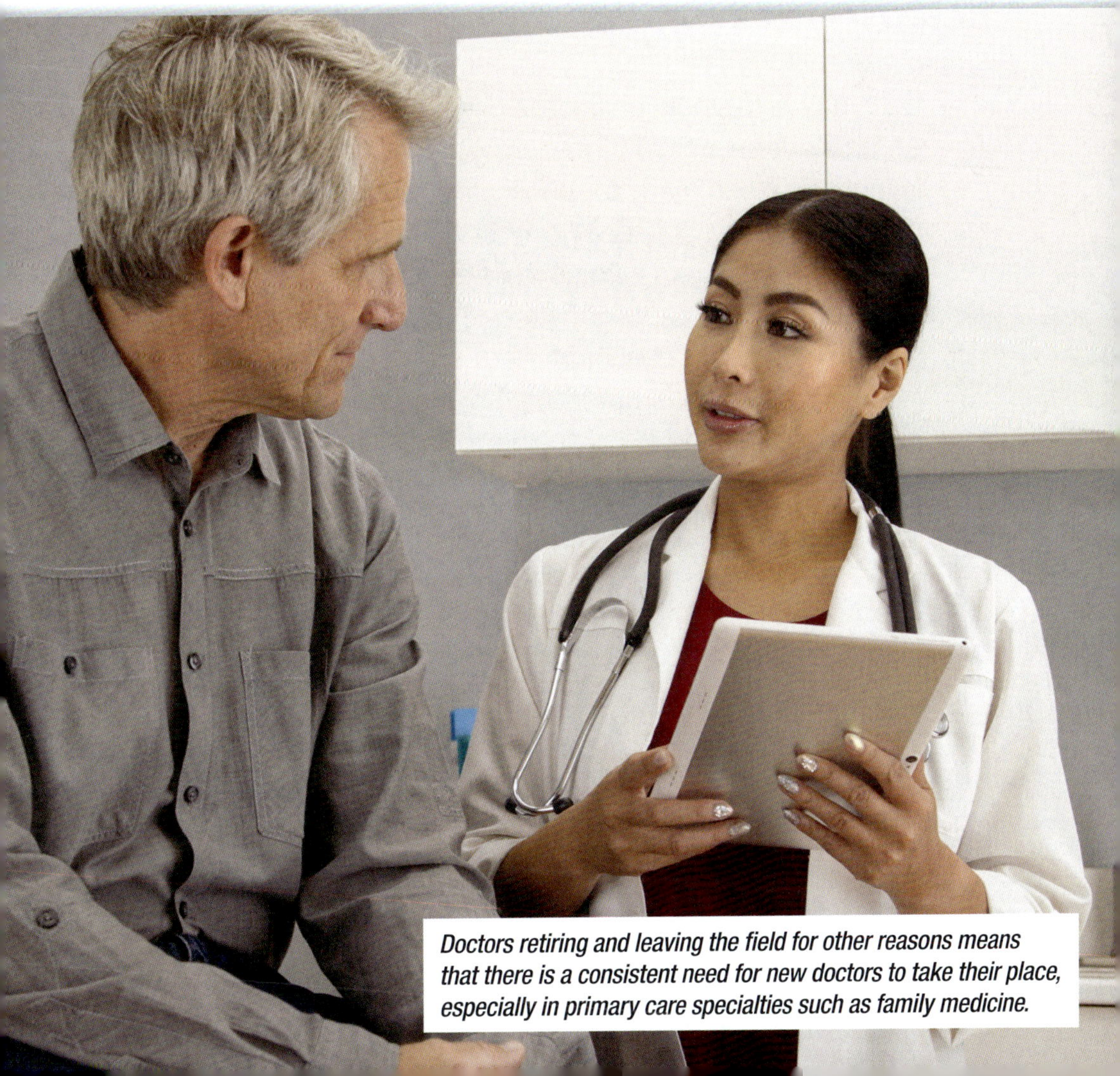

Doctors retiring and leaving the field for other reasons means that there is a consistent need for new doctors to take their place, especially in primary care specialties such as family medicine.

"Each day in this new position is different. I might be editing an article from a fellow physician-author or tweaking the layout of a piece ready for publication. I manage our social media presence and post almost daily on our website. . . . I've also been fortunate to write a few pieces, including an upcoming feature on physician burnout."[32]

—Dr. Jennifer Spector, editor at *Podiatry Today*

Medical education is one option for transitioning doctors. By becoming a member of teaching staff at a medical school, doctors can educate the next generation of doctors. Opportunities in the medical education field also include curriculum development, engaging in education scholarship, or coaching residents or doctors. Medical writing and editing is another job that involves doctors in the continuing education of medical students and doctors. Dr. Jennifer Spector was a podiatrist and surgeon before her transition into being an editor at the publication *Podiatry Today*. She says about her job:

> Each day in this new position is different. I might be editing an article from a fellow physician-author or tweaking the layout of a piece ready for publication. I manage our social media presence and post almost daily on our website. I create e-newsletters with content geared towards docs in my field and correspond daily with current and potential authors. I've also been fortunate to write a few pieces, including an upcoming feature on physician burnout. My clinical background is invaluable to this job, but I have to have a thirst to learn every day. It is a very detailed job, but in a completely different way than medicine was.[32]

The corporate sector—including pharmaceutical companies, health insurance companies, and law firms—also employs doctors. Doctors at health insurance companies review patient records to determine whether ordered procedures or tests are medically necessary. They also are instrumental in determining the standard guidelines for care and overall policies. At pharmaceutical companies, doctors are involved in product research and development, including researching side effects for drugs produced. Dr. Frances

Cosgrove, who was once an ophthalmologist and is now a clinical case manager and medical reviewer for a pharmaceutical company, says, "I've been very impressed . . . by all the continuous learning opportunities in the industry. [And] no more nights and weekends."[33] Doctors also can become expert witnesses who provide a medical perspective on both civil and criminal court cases, as well as in medical malpractice cases. They can both defend physician actions and provide expert testimony about injuries and suspicious deaths to help juries determine guilt or innocence.

> **"I've been very impressed . . . by all the continuous learning opportunities in the industry. [And] no more nights and weekends."[33]**
>
> —Dr. Frances Cosgrove, a clinical case manager and medical reviewer for a pharmaceutical company

Jobs in the public sector, such as working for the federal government or helping influence health care policy, are also options. Health care economists and policy specialists research and propose changes in medical systems across the country. They also work for the federal government and at advocacy

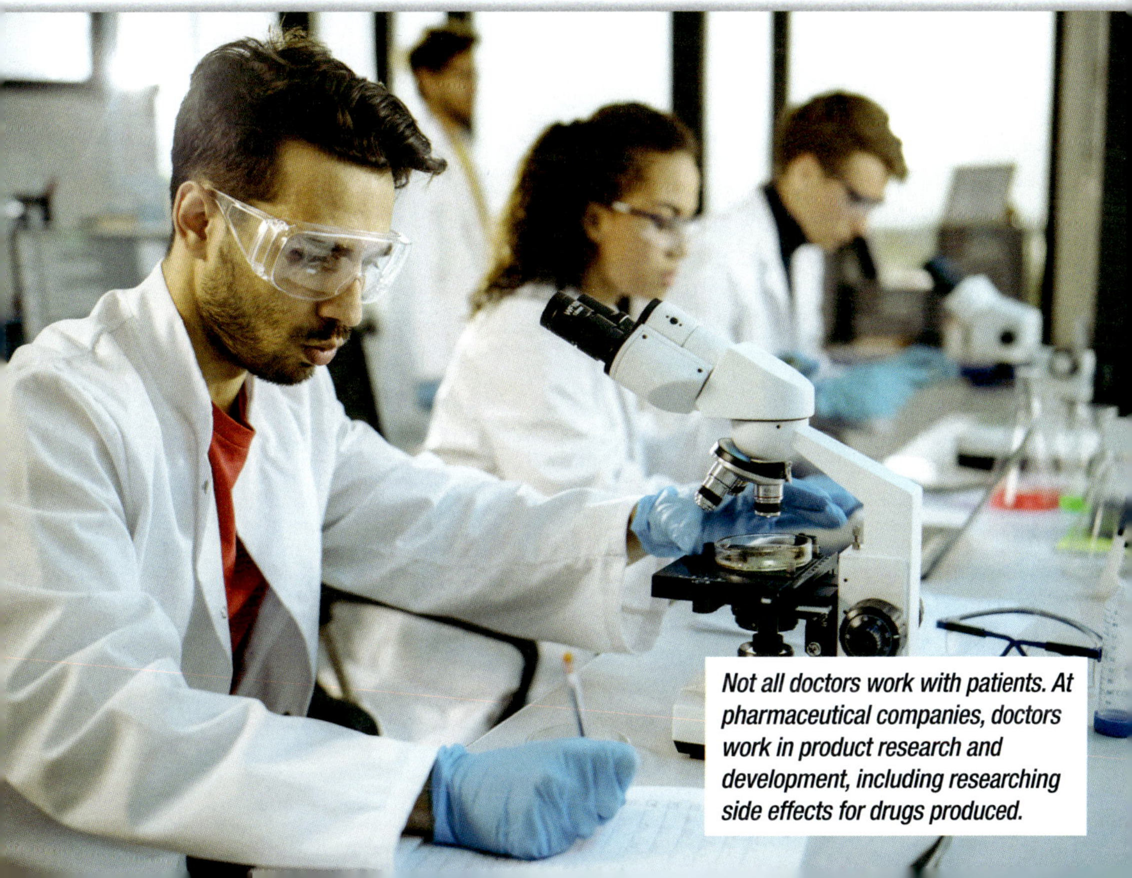

Not all doctors work with patients. At pharmaceutical companies, doctors work in product research and development, including researching side effects for drugs produced.

groups and research institutions to try to identify changes that can be made in healthcare policy to better provide equal and accessible healthcare to all Americans. Doctors can also find employment within federal health care programs as specialists and consultants for Medicaid, Medicare, and Social Security disability to make sure qualified individuals are getting the coverage they need.

Technology's Impact on the Medical Field

It may seem that advances in technology will put doctors out of jobs, but currently those advances are doing quite the opposite. Research into known diseases and conditions, exploratory research to better understand the human body and genome, and

From Cardiologist to Tech Start-Up Founder

"I became a cardiologist and [the] pivot came about, because when I was an undergraduate, I heard a story about an ophthalmologist who had given eyesight to millions of people using a clever innovation that helped him perform surgeries as a pay-as-you-can service. . . . So, now I aspire to live at the intersection of creativity, technology and healthcare.

In March of 2018, I saw a patient with a 10-year history of breast cancer and she was very anxious and nervous the whole visit. . . . She told me that since her initial diagnosis . . . her husband has come to every single encounter. He would . . . take notes and he couldn't be there that day . . . him taking notes meant she could feel liberated to be present in the conversation knowing that they could go home and research all of his notes . . . and . . . go to the next clinician feeling like the main characters of their health story.

[This] is what Abridge is trying to automate for every patient by using cutting edge technology. We can use the app on our phones to record our healthcare encounters. The technology automatically not only captures the audio but also creates a transcript which pulls out the most important medical moments from those conversations."

—Dr. Shiv Rao, founder and CEO of Abridge

Quoted in Gary Barg, "Interview with Shiv Rao, MD," *Today's Caregiver*, November 11, 2019. https://caregiver.com.

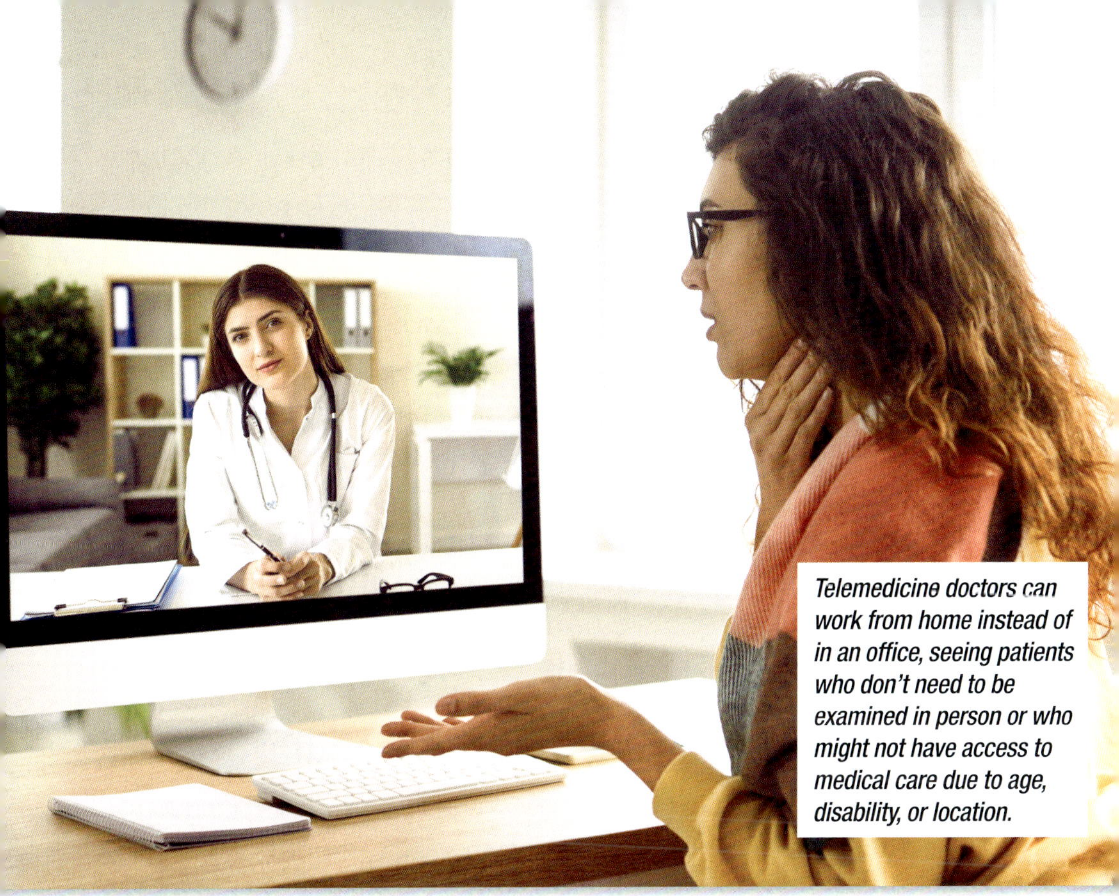

Telemedicine doctors can work from home instead of in an office, seeing patients who don't need to be examined in person or who might not have access to medical care due to age, disability, or location.

development of fascinating new medical devices are occurring due to a growth in medical knowledge and these technological advances. As the medical research and medical device fields continue to grow, they offer more job opportunities for those with medical degrees and clinical experience. Trained doctors are also founding and becoming employed by medical technology companies that are developing new ways to store and collect medical data, building new apps and software, and utilizing new innovations such as artificial intelligence (AI). The medical tech start-up Abridge, for example, was founded by cardiologist Shiv Rao and uses AI technology to assist doctors with taking patient notes and to help patients remember their doctor's instructions.

Technological innovations are also changing how doctors practice medicine. A prime example is the rise in telemedicine, especially since the COVID-19 pandemic. This is technology that can be utilized both by in-office doctors and by doctors who are solely using telemedicine to see patients. Telemedicine doctors can work from home instead of an office, seeing patients who don't need to be examined in person. Telemedicine also offers patients who might not have access to medical care due to age, disability, or location the opportunity to have doctor appointments. Advances in technology in the past twenty years have also allowed doctors to utilize electronic medical charts, communicate more effectively with other medical professionals, review test and scan results, and prescribe wearable medical devices. These developments help with more efficient care and more accurate diagnoses. Doctors of the future will utilize all these technologies and more and are being introduced to their use in both medical schools and residencies.

The Future of Medicine

As is true of many fields, advances in technology will continue to affect the health care field and how medicine is practiced. However, rather than make the job of doctor obsolete, these innovations have increased the job opportunities available to trained doctors and allowed them to provide better care to their patients in clinical settings. Innovations in the medical field also offer doctors opportunities to pivot to other related jobs when they decide not to continue work in a clinical setting. The medical field continues to be one of the most secure career avenues available to Americans. According to the *U.S. News & World Report* Best Jobs rankings, unemployment for doctors is 0.3 percent, much lower than the national unemployment rate, which in the past ten years has fluctuated between 3.4 percent and 14.8 percent. It also is a career that can bring personal satisfaction, intellectual stimulation, and a high salary.

SOURCE NOTES

Introduction: A Demanding Career That Is in Demand

1. Kevin Jubbal, "Why Being a Doctor Is Awesome," Med School Insiders, September 22, 2022. https://medschoolinsiders.com.
2. Jubbal, "Why Being a Doctor Is Awesome."
3. Quoted in Elaine K. Howley, "The U.S. Physician Shortage Is Only Going to Get Worse. Here Are Potential Solutions," *Time*, July 25, 2022. https://time.com.
4. Quoted in Howley, "The U.S. Physician Shortage Is Only Going to Get Worse."
5. Quoted in Bridget Balch, "These Physicians Work in Underserved Communities. The National Health Service Corps Helps Make That Financially Feasible," AAMC, June 29, 2022. www.aamc.org.

Chapter One: Different Kinds of Doctors

6. Quoted in Northwestern Medicine, "Why I Chose My Specialty," 2024. www.feinberg.northwestern.edu.
7. Quoted in Tufts Medical Center, "Tufts MC Plastic & Reconstructive Surgeon Dr. Chris Homsy Provides . . . ," Facebook, June 8, 2021. www.facebook.com/watch/?v=199556848739779.
8. Vivienne Meljen, "Why OBGYN?," sheMD, June 9, 2019. www.shemd.org.

Chapter Two: Becoming a Doctor: Medical School

9. Kevin Jubbal, "How Hard Is It to Get into Medical School? 5 Reasons Premeds Fail," Med School Insiders, March 3, 2023. https://medschoolinsiders.com.
10. Quoted in Claudia Minetti, "A Day in the Life of a Medical School Student," *Michigan Daily*, April 16, 2024. www.michigandaily.com.
11. Kevin Yang, "A Typical Week for First-Year Medical Students," Kaplan, December 16, 2022. www.kaptest.com.
12. Maggie, "A Day in the Life of a Medical Student (MS2)," It's Life, by Maggie, April 1, 2024. https://itslifebymaggie.com.
13. Quoted in Minetti, "A Day in the Life of a Medical School Student."
14. Maggie, "A Day in the Life of a Medical Student (MS2)."

Chapter Three: Becoming a Doctor: Residency

15. Quoted in Wayne State University, "Medical Students Share Experiences as Class of 2023 Marches Toward Match Day," March 12, 2023. https://today.wayne.edu.
16. Annie Kopera, "Day in the Life of an Internal Medicine Intern," Inside the Match, January 15, 2022. www.insidethematch.com.

17. Quoted in Henry Ford Health, "A Day in the Life: Internal Medicine PGY-1," 2024. www.henryford.com.
18. Quoted in Henry Ford Health, "A Day in the Life of a Resident," 2024. www.henryford.com.
19. Quoted in Columbia University Department of Psychiatry, "A Day in the Life of a Resident," August 9, 2023. hwww.columbiapsychiatry.org.

Chapter Four: The Day-to-Day Work of a Doctor

20. Rei Tosu, "A Day in the Life of a Pediatrician," CHOC Inside, March 22, 2022. https://inside.choc.org.
21. Quoted in Lecturio, "Specialty Spotlight: The Life of a Pediatrician," October 2, 2023. www.lecturio.com.
22. Quoted in American Medical Association, "What It's like to Specialize in Emergency Medicine: Shadowing Dr. Clem," January 26, 2024. www.ama-assn.org.
23. Val Vigil, "A Day in the Life of an Emergency Department Doctor," Natividad, August 12, 2022. www.natividad.com.
24. Shailesh Jain, "Never a Dull Moment in the Life of a Psychiatrist," *Psychiatric Times*, December 20, 2020. www.psychiatrictimes.com.
25. Quoted in Emily Henderson, "A Day in the Life of a Thoracic and Cardiovascular Surgeon," News-Medical, September 30, 2021. www.news-medical.net.
26. Quoted in Adventist HealthCare, *Day in the Life: Heart Surgeon*, YouTube, February 25, 2020. www.youtube.com/watch?v=U91AUYttTyc.

Chapter Five: What Skills and Personal Qualities Are Needed?

27. Ross University School of Medicine, "Skills That Make a Good Doctor," October 18, 2021. https://medical.rossu.edu.
28. Kevin Jubbal, "6 Things No One Tells You About Being a Doctor," Med School Insiders, September 21, 2023. https://medschoolinsiders.com.
29. Quoted in Brendan Murphy, "These 8 Traits Make Great Doctors, and Residents Can Develop Them," American Medical Association, February 5, 2024. www.ama-assn.org.
30. Joseph S. Alpert and William H. Frishman, "The Most Important Qualities for the Good Doctor," *American Journal of Medicine*, July 2021. www.amjmed.com.

Chapter Six: Looking to the Future

31. Bonnie Darves, "Outside the Fold: Exploring Nonclinical Work Opportunities for Physicians," *New England Journal of Medicine* CareerCenter, July 1, 2019. https://resources.nejmcareercenter.org.
32. Quoted in Heather Fork, "Transitioning from Medicine—Dr. Jennifer Spector's Story," Doctor's Crossing, May 22, 2020. https://doctorscrossing.com.
33. Quoted in Darves, "Outside the Fold."

INTERVIEW WITH A MEDICAL RESIDENT

Michael Leone began work as a first-year medical resident at Cedars-Sinai Medical Center in Los Angeles in June 2024. Originally from San Diego, California, he attended Albert Einstein College of Medicine in New York City. He plans to specialize in internal medicine. He answered questions about his education and career by email.

Q: Why did you want to become a doctor?
A: I really enjoyed biology in high school and I knew I wanted to be in a career that worked with people, so I was leaning more towards medicine than research going into college. I became an EMT [emergency medical technician] in college and loved it so I knew medicine was the right path. I decided on being a doctor specifically because it allows me to combine biology, working with people, and constantly learning and being challenged every day.

Q: What did you like most about the medical school experience?
A: I would say the community that I was in. I was lucky in that my institution had an incredible close-knit group of students. Everyone was friendly and supportive of one another, faculty included. It made the tougher days of medical school a lot easier to deal with. I'd recommend anyone looking into medical schools heavily consider the culture when deciding where to go.

Q: What did you like least about the medical school experience?
A: Being exposed to and having to deal with the many flaws of our healthcare system was probably my least favorite part of medical school. For example, not being able to put a patient on the best medication for their condition because their insurance won't pay for it, or not having enough time for each patient in the clinic to thoroughly work through all their problems. You really get the behind-the-scenes perspective of healthcare and not everything is glamorous or ideal which is frustrating especially when it impacts patient care.

Q: What was a typical day like during your clinical rotations?
A: This depends a lot on which rotation you're on. Rotations in the hospital, especially surgical rotations, usually start early. I would show up around 7am while on the medicine wards but for surgery sometimes earlier than 6am. I would round on my patients in the morning and get ready for presenting them to my team later in the morning. During rounds we discuss each patient with the attending physician. After rounds we would do the work that needs to be done for the day. On surgical rotations the rest of the day for me was spent in the operating room. I would get home around 3pm most days while in the hospital. Rotations that are clinic-based or outpatient are typically more 9–5. On these I was usually working one-on-one with an attending physician rather than on a team of residents. They would give me patients to see in clinic by myself before discussing them and then we would see them together. Evenings were mostly spent studying for exams given at the end of each clinical rotation which tests you in that specialty.

Q: What were the biggest takeaways from these rotations?
A: These rotations expose you to the core medical specialties so it's usually the time when medical students realize what type of doctor they want to become. You can also take elective rotations to explore other specialties and get a sense for the various environments that doctors work in like the operating room, emergency room, laboratories, radiology reading room, etc. You can also explore less common areas of medicine. For example I took an elective rotation in longevity medicine and I know someone who did an aerospace medicine elective at NASA.

Q: Why did you choose internal medicine for your specialty?
A: I knew after my clinical rotations that I wanted to work with adults and that I didn't want to do a surgical specialty. Internal medicine attracted me the most because of how broad it is with regards to organ systems and diseases. It's a very cerebral specialty and kind of forces you to know a little bit of everything. It

also gives you the option to go into one of the many different sub-specialties like cardiology, gastroenterology, critical care, etc. I also like the option of being able to find work in either a hospital or a clinic or both.

Q: What personal qualities do you find most valuable for someone who wants to be a doctor?
A: I think the most important one is compassion, having genuine concern for the wellbeing of others. Medicine is a service career and wanting to work with people to help them feel better, building interpersonal relationships, and feeling fulfilled from that is what I think prevents most doctors from burning out. Medicine is also a long and challenging career so being resilient is also important.

Q: What is the best way to prepare for this type of work?
A: I would recommend that anyone interested in medicine shadow a doctor, ideally you could shadow several doctors in different specialties to get exposed to the many fields of medicine. I would also recommend being involved in an activity that allows you to work with people in a clinical setting, whether it's becoming an EMT, a medical scribe, a hospital volunteer, etc. Trying to become involved in research can also be useful, especially if you're considering MD/PhD programs or a career in academic medicine.

Q: What other advice do you have for students who might be interested in a career as a medical doctor?
A: The path to becoming a doctor is long and demanding: undergraduate studies, 4 years of medical school, 3–7 years of residency, plus or minus years in a fellowship program. And once you become an independent practicing doctor things might not get much easier, so it's really important that you go into medicine for the right reasons. I've seen medical students and even doctors burn out and I think one of the reasons for this is not having a good reason for being in medicine to fall back on when things inevitably get tough.

FIND OUT MORE

American Medical Association (AMA)
www.ama-assn.org
The American Medical Association is an advocacy organization for doctors. Its website provides information on medical school, residencies, and different medical specialties, as well as tips for mental and physical wellness throughout the process of becoming a doctor.

American Osteopathic Association
https://osteopathic.org
The American Osteopathic Association is the official certifying body for doctors of osteopathic medicine. Its website offers information on the practice of osteopathic medicine for students looking to learn more about the differences between an MD and a DO. It also has information about med school, residency, and career tips.

Association of American Medical Colleges (AAMC)
www.aamc.org
The AAMC oversees all the medical colleges and residency programs located in the United States. Its website provides more information on the MCAT, medical school applications, and applying to residencies. The site also offers a Careers in Medicine area, which students can use to explore whether they are interested in the field, see career options, and choose a specialty.

Health Resources and Services Administration
www.hrsa.gov
The Health Resources & Services Administration is a federal program focused on providing equitable health care for Americans in highest need. It offers scholarships and loan repayment programs to medical doctors in exchange for relocation to high-need areas of the country.

Med School Insiders
https://medschoolinsiders.com
Founded by Dr. Kevin Jubbal, Med School Insiders offers a number of services, including assistance applying for medical school and residencies and tutoring. Its blog also offers a wealth of advice about applying for med school, surviving the med school and residency periods, and study strategies.

INDEX

Note: Boldface page numbers indicate illustrations.

Abridge (app), 50, 51
Accreditation Council for Graduate Medical Education, 26
allergist, 10, 11
allopathic medicine, 19
Alpert, Joseph S., 44
American Association of Medical Colleges, 21
American Medical Association (AMA), 26, 58
American Osteopathic Association, 58
Amin, Ahmad Shatil, 9
anesthesiologist, 11
annuloplasty valve repair, 40
artificial intelligence (AI), 51
Association of American Medical Colleges (AAMC), 17, 58

bedside manner, 44
blood bank/transfusion pathologists, 15–16
board certification, 31
Bravata, Kurt, 14
Bureau of Labor Statistics, 46

Cabatu, Clarence, 29–30
cardiac surgeon, 39–40
cardiologist, 12–13
Centers for Disease Control and Prevention, 7
Clem, Kathleen, 35
Comprehensive Osteopathic Medical Licensing Examination, 21
coronary artery bypass graft, 40
Cosgrove, Frances, 48–49

demand, 46
  for new doctors, 6–7
dermatologist, 9, 10
DeWaters, Ami, 43

earnings. *See* salaries/earnings
editing. *See* medical writing/editing
Education Data Initiative, 21
emergency room (ER) doctor, 10
  challenges of, 39
  typical workday, 35–37

family medicine doctor, 9–10, 14
  projected growth for, 46
Fatehchand, Kavin, 30–31

fellowships, for further specialization, 26
Ferguson, Cara, 22

Harvard Medical School, 17
Health Resources and Services Administration (HRSA), 8, 58
holistic medicine, 19
Homsy, Chris, 12

Jain, Shailesh, 38
jobs
  alternate, 47–50
  numbers of/projected growth in, **4**
Jubbal, Kevin, 5–6, 18–19, 42

Leone, Michael, 55–57
licensing/licensing examinations, 21, 31

Marmureanu, Alexander, 40
Massimiano, Paul, 40
Medical College Admission Test (MCAT), 17
medical doctor
  alternate jobs for, 47–50
  areas most in need of, 5
  general information about, **4**
  skills/personal qualities important for, 41–45
  See also individual specialties
medical education/school(s)
  acceptance rate for, 17
  applying to, 17–19
  careers in, 48
  cost of, 21
  1st/2nd years of, 19–21
  number of graduates from, 46
  for osteopathic *vs.* medical doctors, 19
  3rd/4th years of, 21–23
medical writing/editing, 48
Med School Insiders, 59
Meljen, Vivienne, 14

National Resident Matching Program, 25
New England Journal of Medicine, 47

OB-GYN (obstetrician-gynecologist), 14–15, **15**
opinion polls. *See* surveys
osteopathic medicine, doctor of (DO), 19

pathologist, 15–16
  projected growth for, 46
patients
  bedside manner and, 44
  family medicine doctors' relationships with, 14
  importance of personal connections made with, 5–6

medical students'
interactions with, 22, 23, 24, 27–28
qualities of doctors most important to, 45
specialties and varying interactions with, 9, 15–16
transgender, 12
pediatrician, **10**, **33**
typical workday, 32–34
personal qualities. *See* skills/personal qualities
pharmaceutical industry careers in, 48–49
Physician Compensation Report (Doximity, 2023), 8
Physicians Foundation, 6
plastic surgeon, 11–12, **12**
polls. *See* surveys
Portela, Paola, 8
primary care physician, 13
areas most in need of, 5
See also family medicine doctor
psychiatrist, **38**
projected growth for, 46
typical workday, 37–39
public sector jobs, 49–50

Rao, Shiv, 50, 51
residency, 5, 8
applying for, 24–25
intern year, 27–29
interview with medical resident, 55–57
numbers of applicants *vs.* openings for, 25
standardized exam given during, 21
work-life balance in, 29
rheumatologist, 16

Saad, Michael, 25
salaries/earnings
for cardiologist, 13
for doctors in private practice, 32
for family medicine doctor, 13
median, **4**
for plastic surgeon, 12
variation among specialties in, 10
skills/personal qualities, **4**
bedside manner, 44
confidence/humility, 42–43
intelligence/curiosity, 42
observing/practicing, 45
persistence, 41–42
specialties
rotation among, in 3rd/4th years of medical school, 22–23
variation in pay/job conditions among, 10
Spector, Jennifer, 48
Stolar, Andrea, 21
sub-internships, 23
subspecialties
fellowships for, 26

surgeon/surgery, 9, 10, **27**
cardiac, 39–40
medical school rotation in, 23
residencies in, 27
surveys
on physicians considering retirement, 6
on what patients want from their doctors, 45

Taylor, James, 6, 7
technology, medical, 46, 50–51
impact of, 50–52
telemedicine, 51–52
doctors in, **51**
Tosu, Rei, 34, 35
trauma cases, 36

United States Medical Licensing Examination, 21
U.S. News & World Report (magazine), 45

Vigil, Val, 37

working conditions
variation among specialties in, 10

Yang, Kevin, 20
Yonas, Noah, 19–20

PICTURE CREDITS

Cover: Shutterstock

7: Ground Pictures/Shutterstock
10: PeopleImages.com-Yuri A/Shutterstock
12: Anatoliy/_Gleb/Shutterstock
15: Antoniodiaz/Shutterstock
18: Prostock-Studio/Shutterstock
22: Tongpool Pasupun/Shutterstock
25: PeopleImages.com-Yuri A/Shutterstock
27: PeopleImages.com-Yuri A/Shutterstock
30: Photoroyalty/Shutterstock
33: Gorodenoff/Shutterstock
36: Gorodenoff/Shutterstock
38: Coca Ratta/Shutterstock
43: Gorodenoff/Shutterstock
44: PeopleImages.com-Yuri A/Shutterstock
47: Rocetclips, inc./Shutterstock
49: Gorodenoff/Shutterstock
51: Studio Romantic/Shutterstock

ABOUT THE AUTHOR

Sara Rowe Mount writes articles and books for children and teens. She lives in the Northeast with her husband, daughter, and lots of books.